Hypoglycemia
The *Other* Sugar Disease

by Anita Flegg

Book Coach Press

Anita Flegg
Box 354 Munster
Ontario, Canada
K0A 3P0

www.theothersugardisease.com

Published by Book Coach Press
Canadian Office: Ottawa, Ontario
United States Office: Danville, California
www.BookCoachPress.com

National Library of Canada Cataloguing in Publication

Flegg, Anita, 1960-
 Hypoglycemia : the other sugar disease / Anita Flegg.

Includes bibliographical references.
ISBN 0-9735207-6-0

 1. Hypoglycemia--Popular works. I. Title.

RC662.2.F44 2003   616.4'66   C2003-904739-3

Cover and Graphic Design: Evelyn Budd, Budd Graphics
Editing: Serena Williamson Andrew, Book Coach Press
Workbook Design: Cathy Wylie, The Sharp Quill Ltd.

For Danielle Nahon

Without your help, this book wouldn't be.

Thanks to...

Cathy Wylie, Nancy Lennox, Serena Williamson, Evelyn Budd, Erin and Elizabeth, Robb, and Mom.

I couldn't have done it without your help, support and encouragement.

A special thankyou to Cathy for all your help on the workbook.

Contents

Foreword

■■■■A poor balance in the body's system of handling sugar and insulin is a major factor in a multitude of chronic diseases that afflict mankind. Too much sugar can cause insulin resistance, while chronically high levels of insulin cause poor glucose handling. Knowing that, it becomes clear that any program that improves the balance of insulin and glucose will improve the health of all humanity.

In June of 2003, the World Health Organization (WHO) released a statement estimating that of American children born in the year 2000, one in three will develop diabetes by the age of fifty. Diabetes is already the sixth leading cause of death in America, killing over 200,000 people each year with its complications.

A 1998 WHO study estimated that by 2025, the number of diabetics in the USA will have increased from 14 million to 22 million; in China, from 16 million to 38 million and in India, from 19 million to 57 million—a staggering 195 percent increase!

And diabetes is just one example. Uncontrolled glucose and insulin also contribute to heart disease, arthritis, osteoporosis and cancer.

The people at risk are not just our overweight and under-active neighbors. We all have problems with our low fiber, sugar-laden diet. Everyone is affected—it's just a matter of degree.

We know what to do. We can prevent adding our own names to the diabetes rolls by reducing our intake of sugars and foods (like starches) that readily break down to sugars. So what's stopping us?

We're creatures of habit. We are used to the way we eat. We have always eaten like this and we have been brainwashed into thinking a particular way about our diet and how it relates to our health.

Our current diet is expedient. It is easier to feed the masses with products that have a long shelf life, and in most cases, this means carbohydrate-rich products. A long shelf life makes foods most convenient to sell and store and generates a lot of money for manufacturers. It is sad to say, but in many cases there has been more emphasis on money than on health.

We have been conditioned to accept that it is normal to die in our 60's and 70's. We have come to believe that we should expect the diseases of ageing to affect us as we reach our 60's. There is such resignation surrounding the many chronic diseases of ageing that problems like arthritis, osteoporosis, diabetes and coronaries are accepted as normal.

There is a great deal of controversy around health and diet, and so much emotion and greed clouding the real issues. In addition to the immense profits available to fast food and packaged food companies, there are so many drug therapies for all of these conditions that a change in our eating habits is not in the best interests of many of the businesses that power our economy. Studies and counter-studies abound, confusing the issue and making it difficult for the average person to see the simple answer.

No one can completely escape the ravages of our carbohydrate-rich diet. But simple changes in what we eat can go a long way in improving the entire gamut of the diseases of ageing.

What are the most important changes we can make to avoid or delay the diseases of ageing?

- Reduce our intake of sugar and those foods, like starches, that readily turn into sugar, and;

- Don't be afraid of eating fats (the right kind of fats, of course).

We don't have to accept that we will become diabetic by the time we retire. We don't have to accept that we will eventually have trouble with our hearts. Hardening of the arteries and arthritis are not side effects of ageing—they are side effects of eating the wrong foods.

RON ROSEDALE, M.D.
AUTHOR OF "THE ROSEDALE DIET"
The International Center for
Metabolic and Longevity Medicine
Broomfield, CO, USA

Chapter 1

Starting the journey

■ ■ ■ ■ *We had just missed our flight. My colleague and I had finished a long, exhausting day interviewing engineering students for summer positions with the small, high technology company we both worked for.*

We felt low and dejected so we stood still for a few minutes gathering our thoughts.

"Do you want to go arrange for our flight change, or eat supper first?" he asked.

"If I don't eat soon" I responded "I will really begin to feel terrible."

He looked at me with interest and asked if I was hypoglycemic. I had no idea. I had heard of it in passing from a friend a few years earlier, but nothing beyond the occasional, "Let's go have lunch right away—I'm hypoglycemic".

As we walked to the restaurant, he continued to ask questions.

"When you were pregnant, did you find you needed to eat very frequently?" As a matter of fact, my husband had teased me a lot. "You really have to feed this woman on time", he would joke, "or she gets TESTY".

That conversation was the beginning of my journey with hypoglycemia.

1

Hypoglycemia: The 21st century epidemic

➤ Do you often have headaches?

➤ Does your heart race?

➤ Are you irritable before meals?

➤ Does your brain feel foggy?

➤ Do you feel confused or unable to make a decision?

➤ Are you constantly hungry?

➤ Are you always tired?

➤ Are you worried about taking off that excess weight that just won't go away?

You could be one of the millions of people worldwide who suffer from *hypoglycemia*.

What is hypoglycemia? Well, the long answer will take much of this book. The short answer is that hypoglycemia is *low blood sugar*.

We all know something about diabetes, a condition in which the blood sugar level is too *high*. What many people don't know is that there is another condition in which blood sugar levels drop too *low*. This is called low blood sugar, or hypoglycemia. Hypoglycemia sufferers range from those who continue to go to work, drive the kids to hockey and serve on the PTA, to those who are disabled by their condition. But the lives of all hypoglycemia sufferers can be improved by making dietary changes I will explain in upcoming chapters.

This book will answer these questions and many more:

∎ What is hypoglycemia?

∎ How do I know if I have it?

∎ What causes hypoglycemia?

∎ How can I manage my hypoglycemia?

∎ What are the long-term effects?

∎ How can I talk to my doctor about hypoglycemia?

∎ Where can I get help?

This is not a medical book, and I am not a doctor. I am a fellow hypoglycemic, and I want to pass on what I have learned from doctors, nutritionists, health food storeowners and other hypoglycemics. Dr. Ron Rosedale, a well-known endocrinologist who is an expert in the effects of diet on our health, has provided the medical expertise needed to explain the whys, wheres and hows of hypoglycemia in our bodies.

The word *hypoglycemia* is used in two different ways in the literature and in this book. Hypoglycemia is a medical term meaning "low blood sugar", and just because you may be experiencing low blood sugar at this moment, you are not necessarily a hypoglycemic in the sense that I will focus on in this book. That's because the word hypoglycemia is also used to describe the chronic condition in which you frequently or regularly experience low blood sugar. In these pages, both the immediate symptoms of the "attack" and the chronic lack of energy (and other symptoms) are called "hypoglycemia" and sufferers are called "hypoglycemics".

This definition is, of course, overly simplistic. There are many types and causes of hypoglycemia and it can be very difficult to diagnose. Most hypoglycemics struggle with symptoms and doctors for years before recognizing that the problem is actually low blood sugar. Many of the symptoms mimic other conditions, and most of the tests your doctor will run will show no problem. Patients and doctors alike find the process frustrating.

There are many resources on the Internet and in your local bookstore and all give long lists of symptoms of low blood sugar. All of the symptoms have other possible causes, many of them psychiatric, so it is very common for patients to be told that their problems are "all in their heads". Since the brain is the biggest consumer of sugar in the body, it makes perfect sense that a shortage of blood sugar causes emotional and mental symptoms. The brain simply runs low on fuel.

My goal with this book is to help you discover ways to take control of your life to minimize the symptoms of hypoglycemia and experience good health. Knowledge is power and I believe that understanding your symptoms and their triggers will take away the fear (sometimes panic!) that can accompany the onset of symptoms.

We've all met someone who is diabetic—the primary symptom is high blood sugar. What you may not know is that while hypoglycemia and diabetes sound like opposites, they are really two sides of the same coin. In fact, many medical professionals now believe that hypoglycemia, left unchecked, will result in the development of Type II diabetes later in life. In fact, both hypoglycemia and diabetes may signal problems in the functioning of the pancreas.

This book is primarily concerned with chronic hypoglycemia and what you can do about it. There are many resources available that concentrate on hypoglycemia in diabetics. This condition happens when diabetics eat too little, wait too long between meals, or over-exercise. This is why diabetics are counseled to carry candy—to provide a boost when the blood glucose (blood sugar) levels drop too much. In most cases, this is not good advice for hypoglycemics because the sugar spike causes a continuation or even an aggravation of the symptoms. But more about that later.

This book is not a medical manual. I will not be providing graphic details about the workings of your body. You will, however, learn about cause and effect. You will learn how to figure out whether your symptoms may be pointing to a diagnosis of hypoglycemia, and what to do after that.

You will discover that hypoglycemia and other blood sugar related problems are epidemic in North America, and that most cases are direct results of what we eat. Never before have we consumed so much sugar, thoroughly refined grains and processed, packaged food. This diet is taking its toll on all of us.

It has become clear over the past 30 years that many people are dysglycemic; that is, many people's bodies don't handle sugar at all well. It's been estimated that over 25 percent of all North Americans suffer from hypoglycemia. Most of those 75 million people may have inadvertently caused it themselves through eating too many over refined foods and too much sugar.

If you already know that you have hypoglycemia, or if through reading this book you have your hypoglycemia diagnosed, you are one of the lucky ones. By using the information in this book, you may be able to prevent your hypoglycemia from developing into Type II diabetes.

Take control!

You are in control of your body's operation. Has no one ever told you that before? Think about it. You control what goes into your body and, to a great extent, how quickly your body uses what you put in. Through this book, I hope to convince you that what you eat is the single most important factor controlling how healthy (or unhealthy) you are or become. I want you to know that it is never too late to start improving your health.

Many people, including many doctors, believe that hypoglycemia occurs **only** in diabetics who have exercised too much or used too much insulin for the amount of food they've eaten. Some will never be convinced otherwise. This book will give you tips for getting the medical help that you need if your doctor is one of these.

The internet and medical manuals are full of information on managing hypoglycemia in diabetes, but the following chapters are all about hypoglycemia in the rest of us, those of us who know we don't feel as well as we should or accomplish as much as we would like and want to take control of our lives and live *better.*

Real people have hypoglycemia, too

Many wonderful people contributed to this book, and I'm most grateful to those who allowed their personal stories to be told here. Each chapter begins with a real story told in the words of a hypoglycemia sufferer. You will see that some people have learned to control their symptoms and improve their overall health and that others are still working on it. You will notice that, while there are common threads running through all of the stories, each person's experience differs in some way from the others. Each person experiences hypoglycemia in a different way. Of course, there are variations in the individuals' overall health and social condition, but it is important to note that it is characteristic of low blood sugar to affect each person differently.

Alison
Alison is a university student who discovered the world of hypoglycemia when she was only 15. Passing out in class is definitely a bad thing!

Mary
Mary has been a good friend of mine for many years, but I never knew she was hypoglycemic until I told her I was working on this book. Passing out in the grocery store just isn't normal, either, Mary!

Michel
Michel is a self-described "techie" and workout fiend. He is new to hypoglycemia and is still struggling to figure out what "works" for him.

Laurel

Laurel, another friend of mine, was a big help to me as I began to learn what being hypoglycemic means. She introduced me to her nutritionist and to the basics of the food journal and the hypoglycemia diet. She is a positive and "together" role model and a great support.

Myra

I met Myra online at the yahoo kicksugar group. Myra has been struggling with sugar for years and is now one of the "experts" of the kicksugar group. She's always willing to give advice and help to all the newbies (and the rest of us).

Ann

Ann, a long time hypoglycemic, is managing her hypoglycemia, a young daughter and her business and has just finished writing a book. Although she has severe food allergies in addition to her hypoglycemia, this is one lady who won't let any of this slow her down.

Pete

Pete is another on-line friend who graciously allowed me to pry into his life. Pete and his family have lots of experience with hypoglycemia, and he is constantly on the lookout for new ideas and strategies to improve his health and the health of his family.

Sigrid

Sigrid suffers from alimentary hypoglycemia resulting from surgery. The additional challenge of extensive food allergies has made Sigrid's battle more challenging than most, and she is still not functioning as well as she would like. But she has hope and is not giving up the battle.

Irene

I have never met or talked with Irene. Her daughter generously offered Irene's story through excerpts from her diaries. She suffered for many, many years before learning that the answer to becoming the person she was meant to be lay in changing what she ate.

By reading these frank and touching stories, I hope you will feel that you are a part of a larger community. I hope that you will be able to use what each of these people has learned to help you improve your own life. This book is about hypoglycemia, but even more important, it is about taking control and living with hope.

Chapter 2

What is hypoglycemia?

■■■■Alison's Story

In Grade nine, right around Halloween, I fainted in the science lab and hit my head on the counter. A classmate immediately tried to shove a Snickers bar into my mouth, while the teacher called the school nurse.

My mother took me to the doctor, where I had blood tests and a diabetes test. The doctor told us I was hypoglycemic. His only advice was "Watch out how much sugar you eat".

My older sister, who is a first-aider, knew more about it, and she encouraged me to eat breakfast every day and to take juice for lunch instead of pop.

I can tell when I'm having a bad attack. I get tunnel vision and my field of view gets narrower and narrower. When this starts to happen, I leave class and get something to eat. If I can get something to eat quickly enough, and I can catch it before my view closes over completely, I won't pass out.

We told all my teachers in high school about my hypoglycemia. The science teacher who saw me faint in her class was scared of me after that, and she sent me to the nurse if I got dizzy at all. My

11

history teacher really didn't believe the whole hypoglycemia thing, I think, because she called my house several times to report that I was coming to class stoned. She was convinced I was on drugs because I got light-headed and sweaty and my pupils were dilated.

Now that I am in university, there are new challenges. Life is much more stressful than it used to be and I really notice that my hypoglycemia gets worse. I experimented with cigarettes and pot, but cigarettes make me dizzy and pot feels like a sugar low, so I don't like it. There are lots of late nights and my friends like to go out and drink, so it's really hard to keep to a regular diet and regular hours. Worst of all, it's hard to buy the best food on a student budget. The hypoglycemia is definitely worse since I started university, and I almost passed out in class one day. It was scary, because I was in a large lecture theatre, and no one would have noticed I needed help. I'm sure the prof would have assumed I was falling asleep.

Alison is 24 and a university student—she was diagnosed when she was 15.

Hypo-what?

Hypoglycemia literally means "low blood sugar"—that's the simple answer. The best understood cases of hypoglycemia occur in Type I diabetics. For these people, maintaining a steady blood sugar level, which can be a tricky task, is accomplished through medication. Too much insulin, too little food or too much exercise can bring the blood sugar level down too low and trigger a hypoglycemic response.

There are many people experiencing symptoms, though, and they are **not** diabetic. Increasing numbers of doctors and lay people are coming to believe that hypoglycemia is really quite common in people who do not have diabetes. Many sources estimate that **25-50 percent of non-diabetics** are dysglycemic, meaning that their bodies are unable to deal properly with the sugar in their diets.

In this chapter, we'll explore what hypoglycemia is and why it causes symptoms. We will also look at the different kinds of hypoglycemia.

Hypoglycemia = low blood sugar

I did say that this would not be a heavy-duty medical book and I will keep my word. To understand hypoglycemia, though, we do need a little background.

The human body runs on sugar. Everything we eat contains either a form of sugar or is converted to sugar, which is then used as fuel to run the body and brain. When your blood is low on sugar, the first part of your body to notice the problem is your brain. Your brain uses 20-75 percent (depending on which medical expert you ask) of the sugar your body produces, so it makes sense that a low blood sugar level would affect your brain first.

When you eat something, whether it is a steak, pasta, an apple or a candy bar, your digestive system extracts the sugars and converts them to glycogen. The glycogen is then stored in your liver for use later. Sugar, appropriately converted for storage, also goes into your muscles and fatty tissues.

Insulin is sugar's partner. When your body needs sugar for proper operation, your pancreas releases insulin that reacts to the level of circulating blood sugar and "opens the cells" to release the sugar for use by the body. When your blood sugar begins to drop after you haven't eaten for a while, the liver releases some of the stored sugar (glycogen). If you have a sugary snack (or an easily broken down low-fiber carbohydrate like pasta), insulin is released to prevent your blood sugar from rising too much or to lower it if your sugar level has risen too high or too quickly. A constant fuel supply is critical to proper functioning of all of the body's systems, but this is especially true of the brain. The idea is to keep your blood sugar as level and constant as possible. This is the way the system is supposed to work, but in hypoglycemia, it doesn't work properly.

In many people, the insulin produced by the pancreas is ignored, mostly because the North American sugar-rich diet keeps our insulin levels artificially high, and our cells have learned, over the years, to ignore the high levels. This is called "Insulin Resistance". When the insulin fails to have an effect, more insulin is released. When the cells finally do react, there is so much insulin floating around that the sugar drops suddenly and rapidly. In hypoglycemics, the level of sugar in the blood is pushed **too** low. At this point the adrenal gland sends adrenalin to signal the emergency condition and stops the release of insulin. The adrenalin also signals the liver and muscles to circulate some of the sugar that they have been storing to help bring the blood sugar back to normal operating levels. Additional hormones are produced to metabolize the sugar and block the insulin.

The release of adrenalin (also called epinephrine) is what causes the classic "fight or flight" response. This is where your initial symptoms of sweating, dizziness and elevated heart rate come from. Symptoms can be aggravated if your adrenal system is "burned out" from prolonged or frequent stress.

Other reactions vary widely, but you may find that you are hungry again soon after you eat, or you may crave sweets, or you may feel sick and dizzy. The symptoms range all the way from a mild discomfort to the inability to function normally. In very severe cases, low blood sugar can cause passing out, coma or even death.

My sister and I had our bedrooms in the basement, so every morning I would run up the stairs and sometimes I would end up sitting on the stairs unable to continue up. I would call my sister, and she would run over with a bit of orange juice. After the orange juice, I could get to the top of the stairs. After this happened a few times, I started to take my hypoglycemia more seriously. —ALISON

15

Types of hypoglycemia

There are many terms used to describe the types of hypoglycemia. *Reactive hypoglycemia* and *fasting hypoglycemia* are the two main types of the disorder, with reactive hypoglycemia being the most common.

Many other names are used in the literature describing hypoglycemia, including *postprandial hypoglycemia, postprandial syndrome, alimentary hypoglycemia, functional hypoglycemia, relative hypoglycemia, spontaneous hypoglycemia* and *idiopathic reactive hypoglycemia*.

Most of these terms describe variations of reactive hypoglycemia, and the terms will be discussed and defined in the next section. But first, we need to talk about the hypoglycemia mentioned most often in the medical literature: hypoglycemia in Type I diabetes.

In Type I, or insulin-dependent diabetes, hypoglycemia is a relatively common problem. Using too much insulin for the amount of food eaten or the kind or duration of the exercise being performed often causes hypoglycemia.

In Type I diabetes, the pancreas is producing very little or no insulin and virtually all of the insulin in the body has to come in the form of injections. Maintaining a steady level of blood sugar this way is very difficult, even with a well-regulated diet and consistent amounts of exercise. In the more typical situation, meal times change from day to day, and there is more or less time for exercise as the week goes on. It is very easy to have incidents of high or low blood sugar (hypoglycemia). This is why doctors counsel newly diagnosed Type I diabetics to carry candy—this is the best way to quickly raise the blood sugar. This is not a good solution for hypoglycemics, since it will cause yet another insulin over-reaction, which will result in low blood sugar again within a short time.

Fasting hypoglycemia

In fasting hypoglycemia, symptoms appear when you haven't eaten for five hours or more. Five hours after eating, you may expect to be hungry. After all, five hours is about the normal time interval between lunch and dinner. Perhaps your stomach is growling or gurgling. Maybe you would even describe the sensation in terms like "hunger pains". That's normal. But if, in addition to the hunger, you are having some or many of the symptoms of hypoglycemia (such as light headedness, heart palpitations or difficulty concentrating), that's not normal. (For more symptoms, *see* Chapter 3.)

Fasting hypoglycemia often appears as one of many symptoms of very serious problems like liver disease (including alcohol-induced damage), cancer, tumors of the pancreas and thyroid deficiency. If this is what you are experiencing, you probably already know you're sick because hypoglycemia won't be your first symptom. See your doctor immediately if you think this could apply to you.

Reactive hypoglycemia

By far the most common cases of chronic hypoglycemia are types of reactive hypoglycemia. Reactive hypoglycemia is

17

also called *postprandial hypoglycemia, postprandial syndrome* or *functional hypoglycemia* and symptoms appear two to five hours after you eat. Postprandial, by the way, simply means, "after eating".

When you eat, your body extracts the sugar from your food—sugar is the fuel your body uses to run. Your body works best with a constant fuel supply, so your pancreas delivers insulin to trigger the acceptance of excess sugar by your cells. When this works well, the timely release of insulin keeps your blood sugar at a fairly even level.

In many cases of reactive hypoglycemia, your cells do not respond to the insulin right away, so your pancreas releases even more insulin. This is called *insulin resistance*. This means that when your cells finally respond to the insulin, your blood sugar drops more than it should—low blood sugar. In other cases, eating raises the blood sugar so quickly that the pancreas overreacts, releasing too much insulin and causing the blood sugar to drop lower and faster than it should.

Early Type II diabetes

Reactive hypoglycemia can be an indication that you are in the early stages of Type II diabetes. In early diabetes there is often too much insulin released, and although it is less effective, it often doesn't "turn off" when it should. Under this kind of stress, the pancreas becomes increasingly inefficient and eventually treatment is needed for diabetes. This is why many doctors believe that hypoglycemia should be taken very seriously. Even people who have no family history of diabetes may be at risk if their bodies are under the constant stress of hypoglycemia. The risk is greatly increased if you also have high cholesterol or you are obese. Studies have shown that when patients are diagnosed with Type II diabetes, they have already shown signs of insulin resistance for 7-12 years!

Alimentary hypoglycemia

Alimentary hypoglycemia is also a type of reactive hypoglycemia, and it is caused by stomach surgery or gastro intestinal abnormalities. When the stomach is surgically made smaller ("stapled", often for the purpose of weight loss), the carbohydrates that would normally be slowly absorbed by your stomach are instead dumped immediately into the small intestine. The small intestine rapidly absorbs the carbohydrate and this can be followed by a very sudden insulin release. This can drive the glucose (another word for blood sugar) down to potentially dangerous levels very rapidly. Of all the types of reactive hypoglycemia, alimentary can be the most dangerous.

Alcohol-induced hypoglycemia

Alcohol, particularly when consumed with carbohydrate, can cause an excessive release of insulin and lead to episodes of hypoglycemia. The most common scenario is when you consume alcohol and carbohydrate alone, as with a gin (alcohol) and tonic (pure carbohydrate) and a small cracker or cookie. This is a recipe for disaster, and can cause low blood sugar and its accompanying symptoms even if you never have symptoms otherwise. The occasional occurrence of alcohol-induced hypoglycemia is not necessarily an indication that you are, or will become, a chronic hypoglycemic, but whether chronic or not, hypoglycemia is hard on your body and should always be avoided if possible.

Relative hypoglycemia

In relative hypoglycemia, symptoms may appear when your blood sugar level drops very rapidly. In this case, the blood sugar may not actually drop to a very low level. It is more the size of the drop in blood sugar that is the problem in this case. The new blood sugar level is much lower—sometimes as low as 50 percent of the level right after eating. Relative hypoglycemia is especially difficult to diagnose because the blood sugar level may never even drop below what most doctors consider normal. (e.g. 100mg/dl [milligrams per deciliter] or 6.0 mmol/L [millimoles per liter] is the normal blood glucose level.)

Drug-induced hypoglycemia

The most common cause of drug-induced hypoglycemia is overdosing on insulin or oral diabetes drugs. Other drugs that can cause hypoglycemia are pentamidine or sulpha drugs. Pentamidine is a drug used to treat certain kinds of infections and in preventing a type of pneumonia in HIV patients. Sulfa drugs are used as antibiotics.

Treating drug-induced hypoglycemia is really fairly easy if you know the cause, but diagnosing hypoglycemia, first of all, and then figuring out that the patient has been taking something he or she shouldn't have can be very difficult. In diabetics, insulin overdose is the first thing to check, but often the problem is much less obvious.

Idiopathic reactive hypoglycemia & idiopathic postprandial hypoglycemia

Idiopathic simply means that the cause is unknown, and this is, by far, the largest category. According to one source, idiopathic reactive hypoglycemia is differentiated from idiopathic postprandial hypoglycemia in that, with idiopathic reactive hypoglycemia, there is a measurable drop in the blood sugar level, whereas in the idiopathic postprandial type, the blood sugar levels are considered normal, even while hypoglycemia symptoms are present. For all intents and purposes, this differentiation is academic, and most professional sources do not dwell on it since the symptoms and treatment are the same.

Does it matter what kind of hypoglycemia I have?

Doctors are often reluctant to make diagnoses without corroborating test results. As a non-medical person, I can understand why doctors would like to set a blood glucose level (say 50 mg/dl or 2.78 mmol/L) that defines the line between: "Yes, you have hypoglycemia" and "No, you don't have hypoglycemia". In the case of hypoglycemia, unfortunately, the absolute values in the test results are not conclusive. Different people can have the symptoms at blood sugar levels ranging from 80 mg/dl down to 30 mg/dl and below. We react differently to many things, including blood sugar levels. What one person's body interprets as a low blood sugar level may be perfectly acceptable to another. After all, my car runs just fine on regular gasoline, while yours may require higher-octane fuel to operate well. Whether or not your test shows blood sugar levels below 50 or 60 mg/dl, you could still suffer the effects of hypoglycemia if your brain runs best at 95 or 100 mg/dl. Unfortunately, your doctor may be reluctant to confirm this if she is unfamiliar with the specific test protocols and results interpretation needed to diagnose hypoglycemia.

Your doctor may make a distinction between the types of hypoglycemia. Nevertheless, with the exception of fasting hypoglycemia, where there may be severe underlying conditions to treat, or drug or alcohol induced hypoglycemia, where the cause must be found in order to avoid recurrence, the type of hypoglycemia you have is unimportant. All other types of hypoglycemia are treated the same way—with diet. For the rest of this book, I won't make the distinction between types of hypoglycemia except where the treatment differs.

If you think you have fasting hypoglycemia or if you have hypoglycemic episodes related to alcohol or drugs, please see your doctor as soon as possible. You may need to use the diet information in this book, but you really need to deal with the underlying causes of your hypoglycemia first.

If you believe you have hypoglycemia, and the cause is less clear, read on.

Chapter 3

How do I know if I have it?

■■■■Mary's Story

I remember when I was diagnosed (many years ago now). It was in 1980 or 81, I think, and a friend mentioned to me that it just wasn't normal to be lying on the floor of the grocery store! I had also passed out in the bank lineup one day. I thought it was just the heat, but my friend insisted that I see my doctor. He set me up for a glucose tolerance test. I didn't know what I was being tested for, but I went anyway.

He had me do an 8-hour test and there were a number of folks at the lab doing the same test. Oh yeah, they were all seniors except for me. I managed to pass out at one point late in the day.

When they had me fill in a questionnaire at the end of the day, it asked if I had experienced any "symptoms". At the time, I didn't know what constituted a symptom. I didn't know what the test was for, so I wasn't sure what kind of symptoms they were looking for. The lab techs cracked up when I asked them, and then suggested I note things like feeling light headed, cold sweat, passing out...

My doctor (I enjoy a sense of humor in a physician) said that I had "legitimate" symptoms when I went to see him about results. (This was at a time when the medical community was very skeptical about hypoglycemia and the requirements to diagnose it were very stringent.)

"Symptoms of what?" I said. He was surprised, and he said it looked like I had hypoglycemia. His advice: lower my intake of sugar, make sure I had snacks between meals, and eat mostly complex carbohydrates with a little protein.

I know that if I don't eat both regularly and properly it is very noticeable, particularly to others. On more than one occasion it has been suggested that "you need to eat lunch now!" with some degree of vigor.

Mary works in the high technology sector in Ottawa, Canada.

Symptoms

I hesitate to list the symptoms because *hypoglycemia*, or *low blood sugar*, can cause a myriad of symptoms, and ALL of them could also be caused by something else. I strongly caution you against self-diagnosis. If you do have hypoglycemia, you will find that your symptoms improve when you follow the diet suggestions in this book, but that does not guarantee that hypoglycemia is your only problem. Sometimes hypoglycemia is caused by other, sometimes serious, conditions that you MUST see your doctor about.

In spite of the previous paragraph, no book about hypoglycemia would be complete without a symptoms list, so here goes.

If you suffer from hypoglycemia, you will experience a drop in your blood sugar level two to five hours after eating. Sometimes, the sugar level dropping too quickly, dropping too low, or even just dropping too much from your normal level can cause symptoms.

When your blood sugar level drops to below *your* tolerance level (different for everyone, and it may even be higher than the minimums prescribed in the tests), you will start to experience symptoms.

Many of the initial symptoms are caused by your body's attempt to slow the rapid fall of sugar in the blood by releasing adrenalin. Adrenalin is the same hormone released when you are afraid—it signals an emergency condition. A sudden release of adrenalin results in the following symptoms, the same symptoms you probably experience

when you have just avoided a car accident:
- trembling and shakiness
- heart palpitations
- sudden sweating
- sweaty palms
- overall clamminess
- inner trembling
- nausea
- cold hands and feet

These are among the most common symptoms that adrenalin is being released. Having these symptoms is not a guarantee that you have hypoglycemia. This is why many people who *do* have hypoglycemia have been told that they are having panic attacks. Aside from the clear symptoms of an adrenalin rush, you may also have some or all of these symptoms:
- hunger
- a feeling of mental "cloudiness"
- pallor around the mouth
- dilated pupils
- feeling faint
- apprehension

If you have some or all of these symptoms two to five hours after eating, and you feel and work better after eating, it is very possible that you have hypoglycemia.

Even when you are not having an "attack", your hypoglycemia will have an effect on your overall well-being, and many hypoglycemics report these chronic problems:
- constant fatigue or exhaustion
- headaches or migraines

▌ dizziness

▌ blurred or double vision

▌ ringing in the ears

▌ faintness

▌ insomnia and other sleep problems

Diagnosis of hypoglycemia is further complicated by the myriad of mental and emotional symptoms:

▌ difficulty concentrating

▌ mood changes and irritability

▌ anxiety and nervousness

▌ outbursts of temper

▌ disorientation

▌ indecisiveness

▌ mental confusion

▌ forgetfulness

It is easy to see why hypoglycemia patients are often sent for psychiatric counseling instead of treating them with diet.

Since hypoglycemia is a disorder of the body's ability to handle sugar, it's not surprising that many hypoglycemics also notice symptoms around food and eating:

▌ sudden or constant hunger

▌ lack of appetite

▌ craving for sugar

▌ craving for salt

▌ indigestion

▌ alcohol intolerance

The cravings for sweets are common and sometimes overpowering, and many hypoglycemics struggle with weight problems as well.

There are fairly strong links between hypoglycemia and alcohol related problems, and more than one study suggests that alcoholism can result from unchecked hypoglycemia.

Severe hypoglycemia—seen most often in diabetics whose insulin intake has been inappropriate for their diet or exercise—is an emergency medical condition and must be treated with immediate ingestion of sugar followed by a trip to the nearest emergency room. Symptoms could include:

I convulsions/seizures
I retrograde amnesia (retrograde means getting worse)
I unconsciousness
I coma (This is referred to as diabetic coma in diabetics, but can happen in other severe cases of hypoglycemia as well.)
I death

For the sake of completeness, here are some of the less common physical and mental symptoms reported in the literature. It is unclear whether hypoglycemia is the primary cause of these symptoms, but they have accompanied hypoglycemia in some people:

I pain in the neck, shoulders and back
I muscle pains
I muscle twitching
I vertigo
I restlessness
I unusual frequency of urination
I heat exhaustion

Cause and effect are very fuzzy in the following mental and behavioral problems. It would be easy to understand "feelings of frustration", for instance, in a person who never really feels well and can't understand why. Undiagnosed or misunderstood physical problems also often result in greater stress and uncharacteristic behavior:

- compulsive behavior
- crying spells
- nightmares
- mania (excessive excitement)
- memory problems
- feelings of frustration
- inability to handle stress
- phobias

Why hasn't my doctor told me about hypoglycemia?

There are many reasons why hypoglycemia is rarely diagnosed and even more rarely treated. As a start, doctors seem to have difficulty actually believing that hypoglycemia is a possible cause of the symptoms. Then there is the difficulty in both testing and then interpreting the test. Further, once you have been diagnosed with hypoglycemia, you may still not get the treatment you need since, according to all of the sources, the best treatment is a change in diet and most doctors simply aren't trained in nutrition.

Difficulty of diagnosis

Hypoglycemia is difficult to diagnose, and the range of symptoms you may have will often send your doctor off on other trails. Medical diagnosis is a very complex art/science and it is often difficult to separate causes from effects, symptoms from diseases.

If you have given your doctor a head start by mentioning that you think you might be hypoglycemic, you may still not get a diagnosis. Many doctors believe that hypoglycemia is rare in non-diabetics and that the only way you would have it is with the presence of tumors or liver disease.

This is understandable given the medical literature. According to *The Family Guide to Health Problems*, by Dr. A.-H. Dandavino and Dr. William Hogg, hypoglycemia is a "relatively uncommon problem", and symptoms are often attributable to Dysautonomia or panic attacks, whose symptoms may also be relieved by eating. (The *Stedmans Dictionary* defines Dysautonomia as *"abnormal functioning of the autonomic nervous system".)*

And from *The American Medical Association Family Medical Guide*:

> This condition occurs almost exclusively in people with diabetes mellitus, esp. those taking insulin injections or oral hypoglycemia medication.

> Other causes include stomach surgery, some types of cancer, reaction to various drugs, alcohol, liver disease, pregnancy and high fever.

These are family medical books and not the usual reference books for family doctors, but it becomes clear what the medical profession is being told about hypoglycemia.

The Complete Canadian Health Guide, by June Engel, Ph.D., has this to say about hypoglycemia:

> Tests show that sugar is not a proven cause of hypoglycemia, which is defined as low blood sugar and is signaled by sweating, shakiness, drowsiness, and weakness lasting a few minutes to an hour. Hypoglycemia symptoms vanish soon after ingesting some sugar or injecting glucose, and this prompt relief by eating sugar distinguishes it from conditions such as panic reactions, neurosis and anxiety.

She goes on to say:

> Hypoglycemia is a rare condition; contrary to the popular view that

it's reaching epidemic proportions, it hardly ever occurs in response to foods eaten by healthy people.

With this view established by medical associations and writers, it is small wonder that your doctor may not take your suggestion of hypoglycemia very seriously.

Testing and test interpretation

Even with a doctor who is ready and willing to consider a diagnosis of hypoglycemia, there are more hurdles to contend with.

The Glucose Tolerance Test (GTT), used mostly for the detection of diabetes, is the test used most often to diagnose hypoglycemia. Unfortunately, it is often not reliable as a test for hypoglycemia since the standard diabetes GTT only runs for three hours and often the most important readings for hypoglycemia occur at and after the three and a half hour mark. In addition, if blood were taken at the beginning of the test and then at one-hour intervals, a sudden change at the half-hour mark, for instance, would be missed.

It is important for additional tests to be done while you are experiencing symptoms. This is crucial to make the link between your symptoms and the lower blood sugar level.

As mentioned earlier, often a three-hour GTT is ordered, and the shortened test is unlikely to produce the data required to diagnose hypoglycemia. In *Hypoglycemia*, by Jeraldine Saunders and Dr. Harvey M. Ross, the GTT regimen includes an important reading at the three and a half hour mark, a result that would be completely missing in the shorter test.

Dr. Ross also recommends that a sample be taken at the half hour mark, since that is often when the blood sugar rises following the glucose (or a meal).

Another important test result is the insulin level. Some doctors request that an insulin level be taken with each blood sugar test. Even without symptoms, high insulin levels may be an indication that cells of the body have become insulin resistant. When this happens, the cells stop listening to the insulin, similar to the way parents are able to tune out the loud noises of their children after a while. When the cells don't release sugar at the appearance of insulin, the pancreas keeps producing more until the cells start paying attention. When they finally do, there is so much insulin floating around that the blood sugar can drop drastically. In addition, chronically high levels of insulin are toxic to the body and cause great stress on the pancreas.

Reading the results of the glucose tolerance test (GTT)

Even when good test results are available, many doctors don't know how to read them. Most of the literature defines low blood sugar as being a measured level below 50 mg/dl or even 40 mg/dl, so if your test doesn't show any measurements below these, your doctor may conclude that you don't have hypoglycemia.

The blood sugar level at which symptoms appear varies widely from one person to the next. One person could experience symptoms at 60 mg/dl or even 80 mg/dl while another could show test results of 40 mg/dl without any symptoms at all. In addition, it may be the change in blood sugar level rather than the absolute value that is causing your symptoms.

In *Hypoglycemia*, Dr. Ross describes "normal" results of the glucose tolerance test:

> *All of the readings need not fall exactly into the normal range for the person to be normal, but there are several critical factors to be considered: (1) The fasting level should be in the normal range. (2) Within the first hour, the blood sugar should raise a minimum of half more than the fasting level. Although the graph [may show a] high level of sugar at 1 hour, it is perfectly normal to have this level at the ½ hour reading, with a return to the fasting level at the end of the hour. As stated before, the ½ hour specimen is sometimes very important in determining whether or not there has been a rise in blood sugar level. (3) At the second hour, the blood sugar should return to within a short range of the fasting level. (4) All blood specimens from the second hour through the sixth should remain close to the fasting levels.*

Dr. Ross goes on to explain that anything more than normal variations in your GTT results should be interpreted as the effects of hypoglycemia. A graph of blood sugar levels against time that shows a drop below about 50 mg/dl (2.78 mmol/L) is a standard result for a hypoglycemic. Harder to interpret, perhaps, but still signaling a hypoglycemic reaction, is a graph in which the sugar level drops to around half of the fasting level while remaining above 60 mg/dl (3.3 mmol/L). This is called relative hypoglycemia, since it is the low level relative to the fasting level that causes the problem.

Many doctors will discard any test in which the blood sugar level remains above 50 or 60 mg/dl, and tell you that you do not have hypoglycemia.

How can I tell which type is affecting me?

In general, in fasting hypoglycemia, your symptoms would only begin five hours or more after eating. In this case, as mentioned earlier, the underlying problem could be relatively serious, and you probably already feel sick. Please get checked out by your doctor. In spite of the dire nature of the above statement, you can still probably feel better by changing your diet, as we'll describe later. You should mention the hypoglycemia symptoms and any diet changes you have made when you see your doctor. More information is always better when it comes to diagnosing illness.

If you have reactive hypoglycemia, you are probably hungry or feeling ill less than five hours after you eat. There are many underlying causes, but the symptoms can usually be controlled by diet. If you experience symptoms of hypoglycemia in the range of two to five (some sources say one and a half to five) hours after a meal or snack, and eating makes you feel better, it is possible that you have reactive hypoglycemia. (In some severe cases, the sugar reaction occurs almost immediately after eating as it does for Alison, but this is a result of the sugar spike rather than from low blood sugar.)

Can I take a test to "prove" that hypoglycemia is the problem?

If you have reactive hypoglycemia, and changing your diet works well for you, you may not need to formalize your diagnosis with a test. If, on the other hand, you are feeling ill and are unable to control your symptoms with changes in diet, you should definitely see your doctor for testing.

As mentioned, the standard test for suspected hypoglycemia is a glucose tolerance test. This is a test done first thing in the morning before eating. You are given a drink of a sugary, high carbohydrate drink that you must finish quickly. Then, at intervals, your blood is drawn over the next few hours and tested for blood sugar levels.

In *Hypoglycemia*, by Saunders and Ross, the testing regimen is described as follows:

> *On arrival at the laboratory, a vial of blood is drawn and the subject is given a measured amount of glucose dissolved in liquid. Blood samples should then be drawn ½ hour, 1, 2, 3½, 4 and 5 hours after the patient has the drink. The first half-hour specimen is not routinely done in some laboratories and this is unfortunate since it is sometimes a very important specimen.*

When the glucose tolerance test is conducted this way, the information required to make a diagnosis of hypoglycemia should be available. If the lab has been instructed to take an extra sample when you report symptoms, the test results will be even more informative.

Some doctors also recommend taking one measurement of the insulin level immediately after the glucose drink. Others prefer to test the insulin level every time the blood sugar is measured. A high insulin level could help explain the cause of the hypoglycemia.

Other sources list the definitive test for hypoglycemia as the condition meeting "Whipple's Triad" and is defined as:

▌ *symptoms of hypoglycemia,*

■ *a low glucose level at the same time as the symptoms, and*

■ *improvement and/or resolution of the symptoms with administration of carbohydrate (injected or eaten).*

This corresponds to the glucose tolerance test described earlier, except that it may be even more conclusive because it includes testing for improvement by having you eat or drink at a point in the test where symptoms are noticeable.

With the availability of home glucose meters (used by diabetics), you may be tempted to run the test yourself. Some sources even recommend that you do so. But I recommend against it. First, if your problem is severe, an unsupervised test could be dangerous. Taking a large dose of glucose on an empty stomach and then fasting for five hours could result in very severe symptoms. Second, in checking through state-of-the-art glucometers, I found that most are not accurate down in the 50 mg/dl range. If you have relative hypoglycemia, this may not matter, but if your blood sugar drops very low, your results won't be accurate. Besides, the meters are really quite expensive. Third, your doctor will not trust your test results and will require you to take a supervised GTT anyway.

The best way to approach your suspected hypoglycemia if your doctor is unable to help is to follow the diet suggestions in this book. The hypoglycemia diet is not dangerous in any way, and in fact, is a healthy recipe for living that will work for anyone. If your symptoms improve when you change your diet, it may prove that hypoglycemia is the problem, but more importantly, you will feel better. And once you feel better, an official diagnosis may not be very important.

Chapter 4

What causes hypoglycemia?

■■■■**Michel's story**

I'm an IT techie, I'm in my 40's and I have been doing sports every day since I was 20 (except for sports injuries, but more about that later). I had worked for an IT company for 8 years and I was tired. I tried to work fewer hours for a year but it didn't help. I also had the feeling I couldn't express what I was thinking in meetings and I just wasn't as sharp as I used to be. In mid-2000 I quit working and started some freelance work. For years, I had the feeling that I had lost 30 points off my IQ. I used to be so sharp and quick. But a year after quitting my job, I had lost 20 kg and I couldn't eat without a reaction. It took me half a year to figure out it was the carbohydrates. For a year and a half, I tried to live without carbohydrates. Finally, I found some useful information on the internet with the right search words: "reactive hypoglycemia".

I now think I've been walking around with very low blood sugar levels for years and years. A couple of years ago, I bought a glucose meter. I found that when I feel all right I'm at 4.0 (and I can't get it higher without it dropping later). When I forget to eat or after a workout, it goes to about 3. But I've realized that I have to eat all the time and I'm pretty sure I've had much lower values. Even when I feel OK I'm still not my old self, it's just that my heart is beating normally.

Eating a few almonds or peanuts every half an hour and keeping my meals small helps a lot, but my reactions are a bit different from what I've read about hypoglycemia. Half an hour after eating too many carbs or carbs that metabolize too quickly, I feel my heart pounding like I just avoided a car accident, and another half hour later, my heart starts "missing" beats. I'm also different from many other hypoglycemics—I lose weight when I make a mistake (like eating Chinese food with friends) and it takes about a week before my heart is running normally again.

Since my early 20's, I've done sports every day. The last 12 years I've mainly concentrated on working out in the gym. I weighed 90 kg [198 lbs], and at 1.85m [6 ft 2 in], I didn't look like a hulk but I was athletic. My health was always very important to me so I watched what I ate, no junk food, etc. I drank a lot of coffee, although I wasn't happy about that. Anyway, during my year off, I had time to intensify my workouts and take it easy a bit. But in the next half year I noticed I got injuries in my shoulders and lower back that didn't heal. In November 2000 I went to a sports doctor and he said I should stretch more. I thought it was a bit strange, I've been rather flexible all my life. I did as he suggested, but I only got worse. By stretching, the injuries became acute; the lower back pain was just a warning. The attachments of my leg muscles to my pelvis were severely injured.

From then on I started losing weight fast (I had to stop training) and I remember noticing that my heart was pounding slow and hard after eating. It shook my body. I tried to get back to working out.

One day, I got noticeably worse. After each workout I always ate a big bowl of porridge, muesli and banana, and that's what I ate on that particular day. About 1.5 hours later, my heart went crazy. For a few seconds it went up to about 250 beats per minute.

"That's a bit strange," I thought and 10 minutes later, I was sitting with my head in my hands looking at droplets of sweat falling to the ground. When I looked up it was 3/4 hour later. I called my doctor (I had to wait several days for an appointment!). My heart barely made three normal beats before "missing" beats, day and night. In the following days, it became a bit better, my heart was beating normally during the night but as soon as I woke up, I didn't have to wait long for the abnormal beating to begin again. When I visited the doctor, he hooked me up to an ECG. A couple of days later the result came back: "Nothing the matter— Goodbye".

It was soon after that I noticed that my heart beat problems had something to do with eating and I tried to find what it was. Mid 2001 (June or so) I had lost 20 kg and wasn't very happy. This was not what I had in mind when I quit my well-paying job. Since then, I've been trying to find the cause of my intolerance for eating, or at least a way to live with it. After a few months I was sure the (fast metabolizing) carbohydrates were the cause. And they were in all food! But whatever happened I kept going to the gym. It was about the only regular social contact I had with other people. I'm pretty sure they thought I was a sad case and they didn't understand what was happening with me but I was glad they were there. My injuries weren't healing and I couldn't turn in my sleep or weed the garden. Even getting in and out of my car was a tricky thing.

I was very unhappy with doctors already—I had bad experiences with the sports doctors I had seen about my sports injuries, but a year later, I decided to try one more doctor. "What, your heart misses beats after eating? Impossible!" I left his office that instant.

In spring of 2002, I decided to cut out carbs as much as possible. I started eating vegetables and meat, some milk and yoghurt, and that's all. I knew it couldn't be right but I was punished so often for eating. I had talked about my symptoms with people (even a military doctor in the gym) but they all looked at me strangely. They probably think I must be crazy or a wimp. So I stopped talking about it.

In the summer of 2002 I started wondering about diabetes but when I searched the internet on symptoms they didn't match mine. Symptoms from overdoses of insulin did match but I don't use insulin so it had to be something else. Besides, I thought, if I have enough insulin I should be able to handle carbs all right, shouldn't I? Eating meat and vegetables for meals helped me avoid the strong reactions and kept my heart running better. But I was weaker than ever, dumber than ever and having trouble focusing. And still my injuries wouldn't heal.

Well that's the situation till 3 years ago when I found the word "hypoglycemia" (slow brain you know!) and a lot of what was written matched my experiences, apart from my sports injuries. I began eating peanuts all day and I bought a glucose meter (Why, why didn't I do that sooner?! Oh yeah, slow brain!) I measured low 3's and they should be around 6. Then I knew my blood sugar must have been even much lower for years.

I haven't been "officially" diagnosed by a doctor, and none that I have seen have even mentioned hypoglycemia. But I don't go to doctors anymore.

I've tried all kinds of eating plans but now I eat a small handful of almonds or sometimes peanuts, every half hour. A few cups of milk per day (with chocolate powder, but no sugar, of course), a few cups of yoghurt per day, small piece of cheese sometimes (all of this spread over the day as much as possible) and a very small meal with meat, salad, little bit of whole grain rice. I've tried to stop drinking coffee. I never have smoked and I don't drink, but I sometimes ask myself "Why not?" I see people of my age drinking beer, smoking, eating chips, not doing any sports all their lives, and most of them are still in much, much better shape than I am (deep sigh).

Eating all day (almonds, peanuts, pieces of apple) has helped a lot and my weight has gone up. My injuries are starting to heal and I can almost turn in my sleep without waking up. But I still get too optimistic and I get punished when I eat too much. I'm not even close to living a normal life and being able to manage the hypoglycemia. I still think it's a symptom of something else— something our doctors (well paid, arrogant, uncaring but with lots of status and a Porsche!) don't understand or are not willing to.

Recently I discovered that making my carbs more acid with lemon juice or vinegar allows me to tolerate them better. My injuries have also started healing more quickly and my heart doesn't react to the food as much as it used to. Also eating oats and a specific yoghurt that I can get here work very well.

Not long ago I got a full time job (as a UNIX system admin) and that's kind of a load. I'm very tired from about noon, I lose my voice and I lose about 20 IQ points from the few I have left! Somehow I can't eat enough to keep my energy up, or more like my body can't extract enough energy from the food.

I'm still far from my original strength and weight, but I am improving. Anyway, we'll see what happens.

Michel, still a "techie", lives and works in New Zealand

Reactive hypoglycemia: The diet connection

We are beginning to understand that most, if not all, of those cases of hypoglycemia for which the cause has been listed "unknown" can be explained by the North American Diet. The past 100 years has seen us go from whole grains to over processed white bread, and from water to soda pop. That has to have an effect on our overall health, and this chapter will explain how our over processed and over refined diet has been the primary cause of hypoglycemia, insulin resistance and the mysteriously named "Syndrome X". Insulin resistance and Syndrome X have been implicated in high blood pressure, heart disease and diabetes.

Insulin resistance and Syndrome X have both been "discovered" in the past 15-20 years and they turn out to be part of the chain of events leading from hypoglycemia to diabetes, heart disease and even cancer.

Today's family is always on the go, and shopping and cooking take second place to making a living and spending quality time with loved ones.

Sounds like an ad for convenience food, doesn't it? Does "quality food" have to take second place to "quality time"? Do we have to use pre-packaged foods to meet our schedule? What are we eating?!

Read the ingredients on your favorite packaged foods. I find it disturbing that I can't even *pronounce* the names of all the ingredients I have seen on many "food" packages. Our bodies are not meant to run on this stuff.

We hear a lot lately about the "caveman" or "Paleolithic" diets. We presume that the cave men were not farmers, and that they ate meat and vegetables, and little or no grain. We are part of this evolutionary family tree, and grains are a relatively new part of our diet.

I'm not advocating cutting grains out of our diets, but if grains are a relatively new fuel for humans, perhaps they should be used in moderation. Our digestive systems are well-suited to raw vegetables—lots of roughage, and we know that the whole system works better that way. In fact, studies have shown that people eating a high fiber diet are less likely to develop Type II diabetes.

So why are we consuming mostly bleached, smooth white flour (almost always wheat) and refined sugar? What is this doing to our systems? I believe that the massive change in our diets over the past 100 years is the primary cause of the high incidence of heart disease, cancer and diabetes in the developed world.

Native populations of North America switched to a high grain diet much more recently than peoples of Europe did, so the Europeans have had more time to adapt. The highest incidence of diabetes is in the indigenous populations of North America. Is it just coincidence that the native peoples of North America may be some hundreds of years behind in adapting to a diet comprised mostly of refined grains? The incidence of diabetes is also much higher in people of Hispanic, African, and Asian descent. Again, these are all groups that switched to a highly refined diet relatively recently.

In his 1975 book, *The Saccharine Disease*, T. L. Cleave, M.R.C.P., a retired surgeon with the British Royal Navy, states that "twenty years after refined carbohydrates are adopted [into a culture] there is dramatic rise in dental caries, obesity, diabetes and heart disease, as well as in the diseases associated with low fiber intake including diverticulitis, varicose veins and hemorrhoids".

The addition of refined sugar is another major change in our diets in the past 100 years. The average North American now eats over 100 pounds of sugar per year. That's a conservative estimate—some sources suggest that the real number is as high as 160-210 pounds!

We have been taught that sugar's only adverse effect is on our teeth, and the solution to that is easy—brush your teeth. Other than that, sweets have more calories, so we just need to "cut down" if we need to lose weight. I used to think that, since we "run" on sugar, eating sugar just meant that my body didn't have to work for the calories that I got from my sugar. The truth is that sugar, in its conversion to glucose and glycogen, uses the resources of our bodies. The refinement process has removed all of the sugar cane's natural nutrients, so digestion of sugar uses those already stored in your body. Chromium, zinc, vitamin C, magnesium, calcium and B vitamins are all needed to digest sugar, and these have to be found in your body. This means that eating a lot of sugar can actually result in vitamin and mineral deficiencies.

What we eat has a direct impact on our health.

This is obvious, but we don't think about it much. Most of us believe we eat fairly healthy foods most of the time. Many of us learn about the Canada Food Guide or the recommendations of the American Surgeon General, but we only think about it when the doctor warns us to eat more calcium because we are beginning to show signs of osteoporosis, or more spinach because we are anemic.

According to Dr. Ron Rosedale of the International Center for Metabolic and Longevity Medicine in Broomfield, Colorado, the North American diet is the root cause of most of the 21st century's most frightening diseases, including heart disease, diabetes and even cancer. He has documented improvements in many of his seriously ill patients after changing their diets. Diabetics reduce their insulin, heart patients are able to avoid surgery and patients with high blood pressure and high cholesterol are able to drastically reduce, or even stop, their medications.

Insulin resistance and Syndrome X are the epidemics of our century. As I research this book, I am starting to see more and more information and articles about insulin resistance. It is encouraging to see that these problems are starting to gain recognition beyond the medical community, but it is disturbing to see that the diet link is still in the background. Just today, I read an "infomercial" about insulin resistance in a weekly newsmagazine I subscribe to. Seeing "Insulin Resistance" in a popular magazine really got my attention, but I was disappointed to note that the "article" was paid for by a major pharmaceutical company as an ad for their diabetes drugs.

What we eat has a direct impact on our health.

I am repeating myself, but we need to really understand what this means. It means that if we eat healthy foods, reduce sugar and refined grains and add more variety including more raw and unprocessed foods, not only will we feel well and energetic; **we will prevent disease and live longer.**

Insulin resistance

Most cases of reactive hypoglycemia are labeled *idiopathic*, which means *"unknown cause"*. I believe **insulin resistance** causes most cases of idiopathic reactive hypoglycemia, and that insulin resistance is caused, in turn, by diet and heredity. Insulin resistance can be an early warning sign of Type II diabetes and studies have shown that Type II diabetics may have been insulin resistant for up to 12 years before diagnosis.

Insulin is supposed to trigger the acceptance of circulating blood sugar (glucose) into the body's cells, but over time and with an over refined diet, your cells can become insulin resistant. When cells are insulin resistant, it takes increasing amounts of insulin to trigger the acceptance of additional sugar into cells in your body.

Unchecked, this often progresses to Type II diabetes when your pancreas just gives up after years of producing more insulin than it was meant to. Your blood pressure, cholesterol and tryglycerides readings go up, and you are now at risk of heart attack.

PROCAM (Prospective Cardiovascular Munster) Study: diabetes or high blood pressure increases the risk of heart attack by 2.5 times; both diabetes and high blood pressure increases risk by 8 times; abnormal lipid profile increases risk 16 times; abnormal lipids plus high blood pressure and/or diabetes increases the risk of heart attack 20 times.

Syndrome X is defined as insulin resistance with high blood pressure and high tryglycerides. If you have Syndrome X, you are also at increased risk of developing cancer.

As with almost everything, some people are more quickly affected by adverse conditions than others are. We already know that some people are more likely to get diabetes or cancer or heart disease. And this is at least partly because some people are more likely to have trouble with our over processed and over refined diet. This is the heredity component of insulin resistance. The more refined foods, especially sugar, that we eat, the more insulin the pancreas produces. No one should be eating the amounts of sugar that most of us do, but some people's bodies can resist the effects longer.

Insulin resistance happens when your body has been overwhelmed with too much insulin for so long that your cells stop listening. For the cells of your body, a constantly high level of insulin is just like constant noise in your ears. Over time, you learn to ignore the noise, and it takes a louder sound to get your attention. Your cells view insulin in the same way. It takes more and more insulin to get your cells to pay attention. When your cells ignore insulin and refuse to "open" to take in sugar from your blood, your pancreas simply sends more insulin until your cells begin to respond. The excess insulin has several effects. First, by the time the cells finally begin to accept sugar, there is so much insulin available that your blood sugar drops too much—hypoglycemia. Second, insulin resistance causes more insulin resistance, so eventually there is a lot of insulin floating around your system all the time.

All that insulin makes it difficult to keep your blood sugar steady. When the insulin resistance train has been accelerating on its track for a while, your body really isn't handling sugar properly anymore, and you will have an "abnormal sugar metabolism". One way an abnormal sugar metabolism will show up is in chronic hypoglycemia.

Processing sugar is hard work. Eating a donut or a cookie or a granola bar causes a blood sugar spike that the pancreas must deal with. Every spike requires the release of insulin to get it back under control. If we eat a lot of refined foods containing a lot of sugar, we find ourselves living on the blood sugar roller coaster. Abnormal sugar handling, over time, causes increased insulin resistance.

We know that a high level of sugar in the blood is bad. That's why diabetics stop eating sweets and take medication. A high level of insulin is also bad, but more insidious.

Insulin is not meant to sit around in the body all the time, and excess insulin causes a host of problems. For one thing, insulin is a storage hormone, so if you have too much insulin, you will gain weight because excess sugar is stored as fat. Excess weight is a major risk factor for diabetes, and so is overworking the pancreas by producing too much insulin.

In early Type II diabetes, the pancreas is working very hard to keep up with the demand. Insulin levels in the body are abnormally high, and your blood sugar may be alternating between high and low. This leads to full-blown diabetes when the over-worked pancreas simply can't produce the amounts of insulin needed to overcome the insulin resistance of the body's cells. This slide into Type II diabetes is much more likely in people who are significantly overweight. Sixty-five percent of people living with diabetes will die of a heart attack or stroke.

In addition to Type II diabetes, insulin resistance can cause an increase in blood pressure, "bad" cholesterol and tryglycerides. Dr. Gerald Reaven first recognized that these problems are linked in the late 1980s. He coined the term Syndrome X because no one knew at the time how these problems were linked or what caused them. But it is as clear now as it was then—this combination is a heart attack waiting to happen!

In his book, *Syndrome X*, Dr. Reaven states that Syndrome X "may be the cause of 50 percent of all heart attacks". Syndrome X is also sometimes called the *Metabolic Syndrome*, the *Dysmetabolic Syndrome* and the *Insulin Resistance Syndrome*. Dr. Reaven also suggests that *Insulin Resistance Syndrome* "affects between 60-75 million Americans". More recently, experts have also come to believe that Syndrome X (insulin resistance syndrome) also increases the risk of cancer.

Prevention Magazine (online) has this to say about insulin resistance syndrome (IRS):

> The more of these risk factors you have, the greater the chance you have IRS:
>
> ▪ **Overweight.** Body Mass Index (BMI) higher than 25, or a waistline that measures more than 40 inches for men and 35 inches for women.
>
> ▪ **A sedentary lifestyle**
>
> ▪ **Over age 40**
>
> ▪ **Non-Caucasian ethnicity.** Latino/Hispanic American, African American, Native American, Asian American, Pacific Islander
>
> ▪ **A family history** of type 2 diabetes, high blood pressure or cardiovascular disease
>
> ▪ **A history of glucose intolerance.** A score between 110 and 125 on a fasting plasma glucose test. Or, for women, a history of gestational diabetes during pregnancy
>
> ▪ **A diagnosis of high blood pressure** (130/80 or higher), elevated triglycerides (higher than 150)/low HDL cholesterol (less than 50 for women, less than 40 for men), or cardiovascular disease.
>
> ▪ **Acanthosis nigricans.** These are patches of thick, brownish, velvety skin at the neck, underarms or groin.
>
> ▪ **Polycystic ovary syndrome.** This condition reduces a woman's fertility.

This makes it very clear that whether or not you are hypoglycemic or have high blood sugar, you may be at risk if you have any of these risk factors. Change your diet now to turn back the advance of abnormal blood sugar, insulin resistance and Syndrome X!

Other causes of reactive hypoglycemia

By far, the most common type of hypoglycemia is reactive hypoglycemia caused by insulin resistance but there are other causes, all much rarer:

Alimentary hypoglycemia

Alimentary hypoglycemia is caused by food being dumped too quickly from the stomach into the small intestine. This causes the carbohydrate to be released too quickly, and this is followed by an over-reaction of the pancreas, and over production of insulin. Alimentary hypoglycemia occurs with an abnormality of the stomach, usually because of stomach surgery. Unlike the normal stomach, which can hold food over a long period, the reduced size of the stomach after surgery makes the holding time shorter. Alimentary hypoglycemia can also occur in some cases of gastrointestinal abnormalities not caused by surgery, depending on where in the system the problem is.

The sudden drop in blood sugar can be very dangerous and, in rare cases, can cause seizures and coma. Usually symptoms will appear one-half to two hours after eating.

Alcohol-induced hypoglycemia

Alcohol can cause an excessive release of insulin when it is taken with carbohydrate. Mixed drinks (mixers are mostly carbohydrates and sugars) taken alone or with a carbohydrate snack is the worst scenario since the combination of alcohol and carbohydrate causes a sugar spike. The pancreas over-reacts, releasing too much insulin and the blood sugar can drop very low, very quickly.

Causes of fasting hypoglycemia

Fasting hypoglycemia is the rarest, but most serious form of hypoglycemia in non-diabetics. It is very unlikely that your hypoglycemia is the fasting form, even though it may seem that you have symptoms when you haven't eaten for a while. Fasting hypoglycemia is very specifically defined as the experience of hypoglycemia symptoms occurring more than five hours after you have eaten. Most reactive hypoglycemics experience symptoms only two to three hours after eating.

If you have fasting hypoglycemia, you already know you are sick. The hypoglycemia symptoms probably won't be the most pressing of your symptoms.

The following sections describe some causes of fasting hypoglycemia. If you are experiencing hypoglycemia symptoms five or more hours after eating, please see your doctor as soon as possible!

Pancreatic tumors

If you have growths on your pancreas, they effectively enlarge your pancreas and increase the amount of insulin produced. This may also mean that insulin is produced continuously, not just in response to your intake, so that when you haven't eaten in several hours and there is no food left in your system for the insulin to work on, your blood sugar will drop below comfortable levels.

The cure is surgery to remove the growths from your pancreas. Your insulin production will go back to normal, and you should see your symptoms reduced or eliminated.

Other excess insulin conditions

Other excess-insulin states that can cause hypoglycemia are genetic problems. One example is people whose bodies make antibodies that prevent insulin from being broken down. In this case, the insulin works normally, but it lasts too long and drives the blood sugar down too far. And some peoples' bodies produce an antibody to the insulin receptor, which results in incorrect response to the insulin produced.

Organ failure

Failure of the liver, the kidney or the heart can also cause fasting hypoglycemia as can sepsis (severe infection). If one of your organs is failing, hypoglycemia definitely won't be your first indication—you will already be sick. You don't need to worry about undiagnosed organ failure.

You must see your doctor and follow her instructions and guidelines—improvement of organ function should also improve your hypoglycemia.

Large cancers

Large cancers (non-beta cell tumors) can also cause fasting hypoglycemia. Sometimes large tumors produce an insulin-like substance that can lower your blood sugar. As with organ failure, you will be sick before you notice the hypoglycemia. In this case, removal of the cancer should also cure your hypoglycemia.

Hormone deficiency

Fasting hypoglycemia is sometimes caused by hormone

deficiencies in the adrenal, pituitary or thyroid glands. Deficiency of the human growth hormone (HGH) can also cause hypoglycemia. This is rare and almost always appears in infants and children.

Insulin is also a hormone, and the functions of all of the hormones are interdependent. Treatment by supplementing with the deficient hormones should cure the hypoglycemia.

Drugs

The most common cases of drug-induced hypoglycemia occur when diabetics take too much insulin for their food or activity levels. It also happens occasionally when non-diabetics abuse insulin or other drugs (e.g. sulfonylureas or metformin) normally used to control blood sugar in diabetes.

The next most common drug seen to cause hypoglycemia is alcohol in both alcoholics and non-alcoholics. In alcoholics, fasting hypoglycemia occurs when the liver becomes damaged and is no longer able to properly perform its role in sugar metabolism.

Other drugs sometimes implicated in hypoglycemia are listed here:

▌ *Pentamidine—used to treat certain kinds of infections. Also used in preventing a type of pneumonia in HIV patients.*

▌ *Beta-blockers—a class of heart drugs.*

▌ *Quinine (in high doses)—Quinine is the usual treatment for malaria, and is more likely to cause hypoglycemia in pregnant women being treated for malaria.*

▌*Quinidine—occasionally used to treat malaria, but more often used to treat heart rhythm irregularities.*

▌*Salicylates and other non-steroidal anti-inflammatory medications (NSAIDs)— These are more likely to cause a problem in children.*

▌*Sulpha drugs (sulfonamides)—antibiotics used to treat infections.*

▌*Disopyramide—a cardiac depressant used to treat heart beat irregularities*

▌*Propoxyphene—a pain reliever*

▌*Haloperidol—an anti-psychotic drug*

Treating drug-induced hypoglycemia is fairly straight forward if you know the cause, but diagnosing hypoglycemia, first of all, and then figuring out that the patient has been taking a drug that affects blood sugar can be very difficult. In diabetics, insulin overdose is the first thing to check, but often the problem is much more difficult to track down.

Ketotic hypoglycemia

Ketotic hypoglycemia occurs almost exclusively in children eighteen months to nine years old. It usually shows up in a child who is down with a cold or flu and is not eating properly. In this case, the hypoglycemia appears after a long night without eating and the child will go into convulsions or coma the next morning. This genetic disorder is very rare, and the scenario I just described may be the first indication that the child has it.

Tests will show that in addition to a very low blood sugar

level she has elevated levels of ketones. In children with ketotic hypoglycemia, carbohydrates are not metabolized properly, and the ketosis can be quite dangerous.

Other (rare) causes of childhood hypoglycemia

Other instances of infant or childhood hypoglycemia can be caused by birth defects in the way enzymes are produced, or by hereditary fructose (fruit sugar) intolerance. The first is treated with drugs and the second by avoiding all sources of fructose.

A baby born to a diabetic mother can also be hypoglycemic for the first weeks or months of its life. Being used to the low insulin levels of the mother, the baby's pancreas may be enlarged, producing too much insulin. Often, as the baby grows, the imbalance corrects itself and the child develops normally.

Still not convinced?

By far the largest proportion of hypoglycemia sufferers fall into the category of reactive hypoglycemia caused by chronically poor diet. Most will respond well to a dietary change, and the payoff is great.

When you consider that unchecked hypoglycemia can cause an escalation of insulin resistance and that unchecked insulin resistance can result in diabetes, heart attacks and cancer, making simple changes to your diet is an easy decision. Now that you know that you may be insulin resistant **and** that you can reduce its impact on your health, it just makes sense that you would want to do all you can to ensure that you will live a long, healthy life.

Still not convinced that insulin resistance is a problem for *you*? The 2002 Conference of the American Association of Clinical Endocrinologists was called *The Insulin Resistance (Dysmetabolic) Syndrome Conference* and this was its Statement of Purpose:

■ *To recognize that the Insulin Resistance (Dysmetabolic) Syndrome is an epidemic affecting 1 in 4 Americans, is rising in incidence, and underlies much of the illnesses from obesity and sedentary lifestyle such as heart disease and diabetes;*

■ *call to action by endocrinologists for the public and for fellow clinicians to recognize and treat this disorder;*

■ *define the Insulin Resistance (Dysmetabolic) Syndrome;*

■ *explore the pathophysiology of the Insulin Resistance (Dysmetabolic) Syndrome;*

■ *differentiate between the Insulin Resistance (Dysmetabolic) Syndrome and Type 2 Diabetes;*

■ *define the disease-related consequences of the Insulin Resistance (Dysmetabolic) Syndrome;*

■ *identify individuals at risk for the Insulin Resistance (Dysmetabolic) Syndrome;*

■ *review obesity and its relationship to the Insulin Resistance (Dysmetabolic) Syndrome;*

■ *develop criteria for predicting the Insulin Resistance (Dysmetabolic) Syndrome;*

■ *explore the clinical utility of recognizing the Insulin Resistance (Dysmetabolic) Syndrome;*

■ *evaluate the treatment of the Insulin Resistance (Dysmetabolic) Syndrome.*

If the insulin resistance problem is big enough and serious enough to command the attention of a full conference of endocrinologists, it is obvious that we need to take it seriously, too.

If you are ready to take charge of your life and health and you are willing to make some changes to get there, read on.

Chapter 5

Living well with hypoglycemia

■■■■ *Laurel's Story*

For as long as I can remember, especially when I was traveling or under stress for an extended period of time (as in days and days), I would forget/couldn't/didn't want to eat. I would always get a headache that would range from mild in some cases to moderate in some and severe in several, depending on the level of stress. I would also experience mild dyslexia (I would find it difficult to differentiate between right and left, and would get numbers transposed) and a feeling of disorientation that would get worse and worse as the time between meals lengthened. The disorientation was the worst kind of feeling. I felt that things were out of control, that I couldn't make rational decisions and that everything that I tried to do was really difficult. It made thinking straight almost impossible!

It was when I was traveling with a friend, who noticed the connection between my lack of food and disorientation (I would not be able to carry on a normal conversation, and she said that I had a glazed look in my eyes) that I began to realize that something was a little off. I began to pay more attention to how often I ate but did not pay attention to what I ate.

I was also struggling with weight control and the desire to eat carbohydrates.

After many years of this (approximately 15), and upon discussion with my physician and chiropractor (who specializes in nutritional counseling), I realized that I was suffering from mild to moderate symptoms of hypoglycemia (the symptoms became stronger as the stress became higher). It took a long time for me to make the connection between what I ate and how I felt.

Upon recommendation from my chiropractor and physician, and as I listened to friends who suffered from hypoglycemia, I began to modify my diet so that I always included protein with the carbohydrates. Another big change that I made was to limit the carbohydrates (especially the simple ones). If I could manage to eat protein instead of carbs, I found that the urge (to eat carbs) would go away. The results were really good:

- *weight maintenance is much easier*
- *I rarely suffer from "sugar" headaches*
- *any periods of disorientation that I suffer are few and far between and are much less strong. I have also learned to recognize the beginnings of the disorientation symptoms and can usually grab something to eat before the symptoms get too bad.*

Although my symptoms are fairly mild, managing them through changes in diet has made a huge difference to me. I make sure that the right type of food is available most of the time, and if I am in a situation where I notice things are getting out of control, I am usually able to take steps right away (for example, run into a store to buy nuts, grab a yoghurt) to get things in control again.

Laurel is a businesswoman in Ottawa, Canada.

Can I live well with hypoglycemia?

As must be abundantly clear so far, hypoglycemia is a very complex syndrome that most doctors don't understand, don't treat and which many believe to be the product of a troubled mind.

That's the bad news.

The good news is that treatment is easy and you can manage it yourself if you are unable to find medical help. Best of all, the treatment is without risk, whether or not you actually have hypoglycemia. As I've stated earlier, the treatment is a change in diet.

The diet of the western world is a nasty combination of sugar, refined flour (mostly wheat) and more sugar. One study suggests that Americans eat in the order of 1/4 pound of sugar every day while other sources quote the amount as 160-210 pounds each year! The Canadian diet is very similar, so I wouldn't be surprised to find similar numbers for all of North America.

Hypoglycemia can be the precursor to Type II diabetes and other insulin resistance related ailments, but in less than a year you can turn around the course of your hypoglycemia, and perhaps avert many of the other serious conditions that may be lying in wait. The best news of all is that this diet can improve the health of everyone in your family, and possibly help you all live longer.

Don't be fooled. This is not a weight loss diet. You won't be counting calories or weighing your food. You will, however, increase the variety of what you eat, and learn to enjoy snacking! And, as a side benefit, if you are overweight, you will probably lose weight because your metabolism will begin to work much better.

Is there a cure for hypoglycemia?

Hypoglycemia is a combination of symptoms, and may itself be a symptom. If this is the case, a "cure" would have to remove the underlying condition causing the hypoglycemia. With drug-induced hypoglycemia, this is easy, if you are willing and able to stop using the medication causing the problem. If tumors of the pancreas are causing your hypoglycemia, removal of the tumors will affect a cure since the amount of insulin produced would no longer overshoot your food intake and you would no longer have incidents of low blood sugar.

Alcohol-induced hypoglycemia can be a short-term problem, caused by drinking a mixed drink while eating straight carbohydrate, like a cookie, perhaps, and this episode of low blood sugar will end after the alcohol is out of your system. If, on the other hand, your drinking is chronic, the hypoglycemia is often chronic as well, and following the hypoglycemia diet while reducing your alcohol intake (to zero, eventually) could control, and eventually "cure" your hypoglycemia. Studies suggest that following the hypoglycemia diet may actually reduce the craving for alcohol; so controlling your diet will be helpful and can improve your chances of success in a stop-drinking program.

If you have alimentary hypoglycemia caused by stomach surgery, there is no cure unless the surgery is reversible. If you have had stomach surgery in which the size of your stomach has been reduced, your diet has already changed drastically, and it will be very important to make sure that the small amounts of food you are able to consume are as nutritious as possible. In this case, supplementing with glucomannan may help normalize your blood sugar, but more study is required. More about vitamins, minerals and herbal supplements in the next chapter.

In most cases, the cause of the hypoglycemia is never found. For those unexplained cases, some doctors believe that there is no cure and that the best you can hope for is to reduce your symptoms. Other doctors, often those who have made a study of hypoglycemia, believe that the proper diet, used consistently, can actually improve your metabolism and "cure" your hypoglycemia. It might be argued that you are not cured if you must continue the treatment for the rest of your life, but consider this: would you say your Ferrari was a lemon just because it only runs properly on the best possible fuel?

What can I do to feel better?

The most important change to your lifestyle will be your diet. Since hypoglycemia is an indication that your body doesn't deal well with sugar, the first thing to do is eliminate sugar from your diet. Sounds strange, doesn't it? If I have low blood sugar, shouldn't I eat more sugar to feel better?

The body runs on sugars, and it gets them by breaking down all of the carbohydrates you eat. When you eat low-fiber carbohydrates, (sugar, white breads, fruit juice), your body has to do very little to gain access to the sugar, and you will have a sudden "sugar spike". In hypoglycemia, your body has a tough time keeping the blood sugar level stable, so when the sugar is "used up", there is nothing left and you may experience a sugar crash and many of the symptoms we talked about in Chapter 3.

By choosing to eat high fiber carbohydrates instead (whole grains and raw vegetables for example), you will find that your body breaks down the food much more slowly, and the sugars are released into your blood stream more slowly, too. This will help you to keep your blood sugar stable for longer periods, reducing or even eliminating your symptoms.

Changing your diet

There are many different recommendations for hypoglycemia diets. Some gurus advocate low carbohydrate diets with lots of protein, while others seem to be advocating the exact opposite—a high carbohydrate, low protein diet. In spite of these large differences, the basics of the hypoglycemia diet are all the same. And the first step is to eliminate sugar.

Avoid sugar

Sounds difficult, but paradoxically, once you stop eating sugar, the sugar cravings begin to lessen and the sugary snacks and desserts just look less attractive. Taste is learned, and after a couple of weeks without sugar, you will probably find that sweet foods you once liked now taste *too* sweet, and you no longer enjoy them as much. This is a big bonus, because it makes sticking to the new regimen much easier. It's not enough, though, to forego desserts. Most processed foods contain sugar. Mayonnaise, peanut butter, granola or snack bars, canned fruit and fruit drinks often contain sugar—in some cases a lot of sugar—and these should be avoided as well. When you start checking labels, you may be surprised to see how much sugar you have been eating every day.

What is a good indication of whether or not you should eat it? Ask yourself "Does this taste sweet?" If the answer is "Yes", you should probably avoid eating it or eat it only sparingly. This includes sweet fruit like bananas and watermelon.

Dr. Ross, in *Hypoglycemia*, recommends avoiding everything sweet tasting. His logic is that, to remove all craving for sugar, we should avoid all things sweet. He even suggests avoiding sweet fruit such as apples and raisins for at least the first month or two of your new diet. It is best not to switch to sugar substitutes like aspartame. It is much easier to maintain a sugar free diet if the taste for sugar is gone. In addition, some studies show that release of insulin can occur even with just a sweet taste.

Whether or not you are hypoglycemic, cutting sugar out of your diet will be a positive change. The point of removing sugar is to slow your body's response to food, so that your blood sugar stays more constant. Most hypoglycemics report that they feel much better if they reduce their sugar intake to nearly zero.

Avoid caffeine

Caffeine often improves the symptoms of hypoglycemia, at least temporarily, so it can be tough to remove it from your diet. If you are a caffeine addict, and just can't get through your day without it, it is likely that a sugar stabilization diet will help you reduce your caffeine cravings.

Caffeine stimulates release of stored sugar into your blood stream, so you will feel better for a while but your blood sugar will drop abruptly again once the effect of the caffeine wears off. As my nutritionist, Dr. Todd Norton, describes it, "In asking the cells to release sugar, insulin knocks at the door. Caffeine, on the other hand, simply kicks the door down!" Another reason that you get a boost from caffeine is that it stimulates the adrenal gland. This makes your heart beat faster and raises your blood sugar. Excess caffeine also puts stress on your kidneys, and flushes minerals like selenium, manganese, zinc, calcium and magnesium from your body.

My first response was, "So what—I really feel better. I *neeeeed* it!" Caffeine, like sugar, causes a roller coaster of sugar highs and lows. I know that after I drink caffeinated drinks, I find that I am constantly hungry and it takes me a couple of days of proper eating to get back on track. As you learn to regulate your blood sugar by changing your diet, even your cravings for caffeine will subside.

Quit smoking

I know, I know—now I have really gone overboard! We have been hearing for years that nicotine will kill you and we have all lost people important to us. What you, as a hypoglycemic, need to know is that nicotine affects blood sugar. Nicotine, like caffeine, activates the adrenal gland. Your heart speeds up and your blood pressure rises and you get that much-needed boost. Although butting out may be much more difficult than eliminating caffeine, you will find that as you change your diet and begin to feel better, your cravings for nicotine will slowly begin to subside. Quitting still may not be easy; after all, cigarettes have become a habit based on more than the nicotine addiction. As your blood sugar begins to stabilize, you will find that it will be easier to taper down to fewer cigarettes per day.

Avoid alcohol

Alcohol, like sugar, contains nothing but calories. It has no nutritive value at all and moves very quickly into your blood stream. This affects your blood sugar very suddenly, and there is a corresponding drop in blood sugar as the alcohol leaves your system.

The problem of maintaining a constant blood sugar level is common to both hypoglycemics and diabetics. For diabetics, the insulin injected must compensate for the food and drink consumed. An old friend of mine, an insulin dependent diabetic, once told me why he avoids alcohol.

Roy said:

> It's a challenge to figure out how much insulin I will need to match my food intake and the amount of exercise I do. I have a routine that includes a standard, no sugar diet, and lots of exercise every day. I plan my food so that I eat the same amounts at the same times of day, and I get my bike out for an hour every evening. And

I don't drink— it's just too difficult to get the insulin right to compensate for it.

In diabetes, you can control your sugar level with injected insulin. In hypoglycemia this is not possible, and if you eat and drink foods that play havoc with your blood sugar level, you just have to live with the symptoms. It's much better then, to avoid the booze and the feeling rotten that comes with it.

An extra caution: Read the labels on all your medications; many include alcohol. You need to find alternatives if at all possible. Talk to your doctor or pharmacist if you have prescription medication containing alcohol, and ask for help finding an alcohol-free alternative. Some allergy shots also contain alcohol, so check with your doctor.

Switch to high fiber carbohydrates

All foods sit on a continuum that relates their sugar content to how fast they are used in your body. This is called the glycemic index. We'll explore this more in another chapter, but for now, we'll just note that high fiber foods are low on the glycemic index.

In order to keep your blood sugar constant with as few peaks and valleys as possible, you need to slow the rate at which your body converts your food to the various kinds of sugar used and stored in your body. The best way to do this is to eat foods that, in addition to supplying all the right components of nutrition, burn very slowly.

Since the goal is to slow the rate at which your food is broken down, it is important to avoid fast burning, high glycemic foods starting with sugar, but also including refined foods. This includes white flour, white rice, and other refined and polished grains.

The breads category of your new diet will include only whole grain breads, brown rice, and other grains such as quinoa and millet—high fiber carbohydrates. Lots of vegetables will fill out the balance of your intake with the occasional piece of fruit added for variety.

When you eat fruit and vegetables, eat them raw and with the skin as often as you can. Peeling removes much of the fiber and many of the vitamins and minerals, and cooking results in the loss of most of the vitamins into the water.

Even potatoes, a staple for most of us, should be used in moderation only. Try switching to sweet potatoes for variety—believe or not, sweet potatoes actually break down more slowly than ordinary white potatoes. The "sweet" in sweet potato seems to be a misnomer!

Choose balanced snacks and meals

When my daughter was diagnosed with low blood sugar many years ago (on the basis of one blood sample!) the advice of the doctor was simply this *"Make sure she eats protein with every meal and snack."* I have followed this advice for myself and both of my children ever since and I have found that for myself and for my hypoglycemic daughter, this makes a huge difference. Where I used to snack on an apple, I began adding a small piece of cheddar cheese. Instead of a cookie, I would give my daughter yogurt. When she was diagnosed, she was in a "chicken noodle soup phase" and that is all she would eat, so I added small amounts of diced, cooked chicken.

I have found that the most effective meals and snacks, effective being the measure of how I felt and how long before I was hungry again, contain moderate amounts of protein, carbohydrate and fat. Protein, like high fiber carbohydrates, takes time and effort to break down.

Here are some good snacks that contain all three:

- Nuts; raw and unsalted (no peanuts – at least for the first few months)
- Whole grain crackers with nut butter (cashew butter or almond butter)
- Whole wheat pita bread or whole grain crackers with hummus (a mixture of chick peas, sesame seed paste and garlic)
- Whole grain crackers with avocado and a dash of salt and lemon juice. Avocado is a wonderful food for hypoglycemics because it is a source of many essential fatty acids plus beneficial vitamins and minerals.
- A tofu or protein shake with berries
- A small salad (not iceberg lettuce) with cheese and sunflower seeds
- Sardines
- Raw vegetables like celery, cucumber or broccoli with a protein dip like almond or cashew butter, cream cheese or tuna salad. Hummus or smoked fish or sardines mixed with cream cheese also make good dips.

In all of these examples, there is a good balance of protein, carbohydrate and fat, and all of them will lengthen the time before you need to eat again. Before I started the hypoglycemia diet, I was hungry almost all the time and it really affected my ability to concentrate. After learning to snack properly, I now find that I can really get down to work and not think about food all the time.

Not all of these snack suggestions will work for you—experimentation will tell you which snacks are most satisfying and long lasting. Keep in mind, too, that some of these foods may also cause allergic reactions. Experts say that the top allergens are wheat, corn and dairy, and of course, peanuts, and you may not even know you are sensitive to these foods unless you stop eating them for a while. Allergies and food sensitivities are common in hypoglycemics, and we will explore the subject of hypoglycemia and allergies in a later chapter.

Eat small amounts frequently

If you are hypoglycemic, you may feel hungry more often than many of your friends and family do. Follow your appetite. If you find that you begin to be hungry, or you often feel unwell about three hours after a meal or snack, plan to eat every two and a half hours. If you have symptoms two hours after eating, plan your snacks and meals to occur at one and a half hour intervals.

Even when you feel very hungry, stick to small meals and snacks. You may find that the amount of food you eat really doesn't affect how long you can go before you need to eat again, so eating more than just enough to satisfy you will lead to weight gain.

As your metabolism changes, you should find that you are able to increase the intervals—just make sure you continue to eat nutritious, high fiber carbohydrates with proteins and fats.

Keep in mind that the three-meal-a-day model will probably never work for you. Some people may be able to tolerate it, but everyone would probably function better with more small meals. What you **will** be able to do is wait for a meal or skip a snack occasionally without the serious symptoms you experience now.

Get enough sleep

The number of hours of sleep needed varies from person to person, but not as much as you might think. Some people like to brag that they only need four or five hours of sleep per night. I, myself, have expressed the opinion on more than one occasion that sleep is a real waste of time—there just aren't enough hours in a day for me to want to "waste" eight of them unconscious.

The truth is, though, that no one should imagine that they can function on less than about seven or seven and a half hours of sleep per night. Sleep is the time your body uses to replenish and rebuild. When you are low on sleep your body will have a tougher time coping with a less-than-perfect diet. Constantly running a sleep deficit, something most of us do at least occasionally, can really lower your body's ability to rebuild and to keep your immune system strong.

Lower the stress in your life

Easy to say, hard to do.

Stress aggravates many medical conditions and low blood sugar is one of them. If you work long hours and feel a great deal of stress at work, low blood sugar symptoms seem to come on more quickly and the symptoms seem to be worse.

Of all of the changes I'm asking you to make, reducing the stress in your life may be the hardest because the amount of stress you deal with is directly related to the lifestyle you have chosen (or have had chosen for you). There are many stressful things in your life that you won't be able to change. You won't be able to change the fact that you are a single parent with a full-time job. You can't do anything to change the fact that someone close to you has just died, either, but there are many things that you can do to reduce the stress in your life.

The first thing to change is how you see the stress. Your stress level will be much higher if you feel overwhelmed. Take some time to look carefully at the stressors in your life. List them if you need to. Then think about one thing you can do that will reduce stress in one aspect of your life. That one, simple, positive act will already make you feel better because you will no longer feel powerless.

Sometimes (and I have definitely been there) the stress is so overwhelming that you can't even see that there may be choices you could make to reduce your stress.

Take the example of single parenthood and that full-time job, for instance. You have kids—you can't change that—and you have to work full-time to make ends meet. This is a perfect example of a high stress lifestyle. You may think that there is nothing you can do about it, but there may be a few changes you could make that would take away that out-of-control feeling and help lower your stress. Do you like your job? If you don't, your job is a huge source of stress. Try to find a job you will enjoy. You still have to work full-time, but you will have one less source of stress in your life.

Don't be ashamed to ask for help. Independence and self-sufficiency can be taken to a stressful extreme. There are people around you who care about you and who would like to help if you would only ask. Let them take the kids for the afternoon or cook you a meal. I guarantee you will feel better if you loosen the reins on yourself a bit.

This takes practice, but it gets easier. Try it—both your mind and your body will thank you.

Exercise

Exercise is an important component in the management of hypoglycemia because it is a great metabolic booster. Increased insulin sensitivity and lower insulin needs are some of its benefits along with improved glucose tolerance. Exercise can also reduce cholesterol and tryglyceride levels.

Hypoglycemics often carry high amounts of insulin all the time. Insulin affects the production and use of estrogen, so if your insulin is always too high, you are more likely to have more bone loss than you should for your age.

In addition to changing your diet to get your insulin and blood sugar under control, starting a weight-training program is one of the best things you can do to improve your health. In addition to toning and strengthening your muscles, it can help slow down the process of osteoporosis by putting (good) stress on your bones. Join a gym or buy some inexpensive weights and get a partner. It is always easier (and more fun) to stick to a lifestyle change if you have someone to share it with. Hire a trainer to help you develop a program. It doesn't have to be expensive. If you prefer, buy a good weight training manual. There are many great books to show you proper positions that will work the desired muscles and prevent injury. Start with your largest muscles. This will give you the quickest results because the large muscles burn more calories. Begin with low weight and increase repetitions until even 30 or 40 repetitions are easy to complete. Then you can increase the weight. This isn't a quick fix, but working out with weights two or three times per week will make a difference to how you look and feel.

Aerobic exercise is important for improved health and well-being, and improves fat burning. Humans are meant to move, and raising your heart rate pushes the capability of your lungs and heart, improving oxygen processing in your lungs and strengthening your heart. You don't need to train for a marathon to see the benefits of aerobic exercise. A brisk walk three to five times a week will do very well. Take your kids, your spouse, your dog—it should be fun. Or get out your bike. Cycling is a great way to get your exercise and enjoy the sights.

It is well documented that exercise increases endorphins, creating a natural "high". That's the effect we see when we become "addicted" to exercise. We all know that exercise increases calorie burning and promotes weight loss—important for your overall health. Feeling great, both physically and mentally, really helps you stay motivated in the rest of your lifestyle changes. Just remember to take a snack with you—when you exercise, you will need to eat sooner.

If I'm hypoglycemic, does that mean that I will always be overweight?

Insulin is a storage chemical, so if your body is producing too much insulin, chances are you will carry too much weight. This isn't a hard and fast rule, though. Some hypoglycemics are underweight and just can't gain weight.

The excess insulin is why it is very difficult for many hypoglycemics to lose weight. Using the diet recommendations in this book, you will begin to stabilize your blood sugar, and by extension, your insulin production. Once this improvement to your metabolism begins, many of your other hormones will start to normalize, too. This will change your body's set point, and you should drift slowly down to your proper weight. This will be a slow process, and you should not count calories or become obsessed with your weight. Instead, continue to concentrate on improving your well-being through eating well.

The National Weight Control Registry

Jim Hill, PhD, of the University of Colorado, noticed that there are very few people who are able to lose weight and keep it off for at least a year. He started the National Weight Control Registry to track the people who succeeded in losing at least 30 pounds and kept it off for at least a year.

Information and case studies appeared on CNN on July 6, 2002 on a program called "Fat Chance" with medical correspondent Elizabeth Cohen.

Of all the things these "club members" do to maintain their lower, healthier weights, there are seven things that all of the participants have in common. Keep in mind that there are additional constraints for the hypoglycemic diet, but most of these are great advice for hypoglycemics as well.

1. **Expect failure, but keep trying.** Most of the Registry participants made the decision to lose weight because of fear for their health. Motivation like this makes it easier to stick to your plan because everything you eat or don't eat is a conscious decision based on your priorities. If improving your health through weight loss is a high priority in your life, your eating (and exercise) decisions will reflect this, not just today, but over the long term. [Sticking to your hypoglycemic diet should also reflect a personal health decision since I believe that getting your blood sugar under control now can reduce the risk of many serious health problems! Don't expect perfection—just keep trying.]

2. **Don't deny yourself.** Feeling deprived is why you binge. Rather than completely eliminating all of the so-called "bad foods", try to keep it to a taste instead of a whole helping, have just one spoonful of the foods you crave. [Keep in mind that even a small amount of sugar can cause symptoms and setbacks for a hypoglycemic, so don't cheat on the sugar, at least for the first few months.]

3. **Weigh yourself often.** Motivation, motivation, motivation! [Your primary concern should be improving your general health, but if watching your weight fall motivates you to stick to the diet, do it.]

4. **Plan at least an hour a day of serious exercise.** In addition to making you feel energized and terrific, aerobic exercise helps increase your metabolic rate, and you will use calories faster. Adding some weight lifting will increase your muscle mass, and muscle burns more calories than fat. Improving your muscle tone will also make your daily activities easier. [Great for hypoglycemics and non-hypoglycemics alike.]

5. **Add little bits of activity throughout your daily routine.** Park at the far end of the lot; take the stairs; walk over to your neighbor's house rather than calling on the phone; walk to the corner store for milk rather than driving—and then turn all of these changes into habits. [Saves the environment, too.]

6. **Eat a high carbohydrate, low fat diet.** Not all of the experts would agree on this, but most of the participants in this Registry have increased their carbs and reduced their fat intake. [A lower carbohydrate, higher protein diet is often very successful for hypoglycemics.]

7. **Eat at least five times each day and don't skip breakfast.** Just goes to show, this works for hypoglycemics and non-hypoglycemics as well. The theory is that if you eat small amounts often, you will be less tempted to overeat. For those of us who are hypoglycemic, this survival skill may actually help us lose weight in addition to reducing symptoms.

Chapter 6

What supplements should I take?

While I don't know for sure, I bet that I was hypoglycemic ever since I was a young child. I know I have been a sugar addict since I was very young.

I recall several Saturday mornings when I was up early to watch cartoons. I immediately started eating dry, highly sweetened breakfast cereals—Sugar Pops, Sugar Smacks, Frosted Flakes, etc. and candy while lying on the living room couch. When I got up to do something, I remember blacking out or nearly blacking out. My mother said it was because I got up too quickly, but I know now that it was likely a hypoglycemic reaction from all that sugary food I was eating.

Sugar was just a way of life for me. Not just sugary cereal, but pancakes with loads of maple syrup, cookies, cakes, chocolates and on and on. It is amazing to me that my parents fed me all these sugary treats along with a ton of highly refined food—pasta, white rice, TV dinners, white bread sandwiches—considering that there was an overwhelmingly amount of diabetes in my family. My dad's father died from insulin shock. I had aunts, uncles and first cousins who were all diabetics. My dad was borderline diabetic as well. I guess they just never made the connection between the sugar and the tendency toward diabetes. Our doctors never said anything about this, either.

Looking back I had a number of hypo symptoms. I was a very moody and depressed child and teenager. I remember seriously considering committing suicide when I was about 13. I cried all the time. I was tired all the time. I had all kinds of headaches—debilitating ones that kept me out of school. I was totally uncoordinated. I had bad insomnia. I had blurred vision. My parents took me to the doctor when I was in high school for the blurred vision. They did an EEG, but didn't find anything. They figured it was nerves, especially since my mother was also very, very nervous (sometimes I wonder if she has hypoglycemia too, but she has never had it checked and probably never will).

I never gave these symptoms a second thought and I just kept on eating sugar and other refined carbs in huge quantities on a regular basis. I remember many occasions that I practically emptied a whole can of ready-made frosting and no cake or candy was safe from me. I would make my husband go to the corner deli and buy an Entenmann's Chocolate Blackout Cake (chocolate cake filled with chocolate pudding, yum!) and within an hour we both devoured the whole cake. It was largely my doing as my husband is much more a salty than a sweet snacker.

I hit bottom about two years after my son was born. It was sometime around Easter and I went over to my in-laws' house. They had all kinds of Easter candies out. Needless to say, I ate a whole lot of candy and shortly after I did, I found myself on the floor of my mother-in-law's kitchen, right next to the refrigerator with my husband leaning over me making sure I was okay. It was really scary.

The next week I went to one doctor, who was unconcerned that I passed out. My husband, who had read something about hypoglycemia realized it fit me to a "T"—not just my passing out but also my moodiness, extreme tiredness and depression, suggested to him that he give me a glucose tolerance test. He refused. A friend of ours suggested another doctor to see—actually a physician's assistant. We told him our concerns and he was more receptive to our suggestions. He did first want to run another test, which came out negative and then gave me a five-hour glucose tolerance test. He had to interrupt the test before the five hours were up because my blood sugar (which tested normal in a regular fasting blood test) fell so far down. He said I was perhaps the worst case of a reactive hypoglycemic that he had ever seen. He gave me something to get my blood sugar back up, told me to eat some protein as soon as I got home (making sure my husband would drive), told me to not have anything with any sugar in it and to make an appointment with a registered dietitian (he gave me the name of one).

The next few days were pure hell. I was shaking from the sugar withdrawal. I felt like I was on a roller coaster ride. I know I wouldn't have made it through the terrible withdrawal symptoms without my husband's support. He stayed beside me and comforted me and held my hand. He was great.

When I went to the dietitian she came up with an eating program that helped somewhat. She concurred that I needed to stay away from sugars, but didn't have me stay from other refined carbs, which I now realize I should have done. She put me on a diabetic diet (in fact she handed me a brochure from the American Diabetic Association). But stopping eating sugar and eating frequently helped me some. It took a while, but eventually I was totally symptom free as long as I didn't wait too long to eat and didn't have sweet foods. I must admit that I wasn't 100 percent perfect, every now and then treating myself to a small dessert on a special occasion, but it was amazing how much better I felt and how it made my husband happier not having to deal with my crazy highs and lows, mainly lows.

I remained fairly symptom free for many years until about three years ago. I don't know what caused the change. It could have been all the stress in our lives—money problems, my son having extreme problems in school, our landlord selling our house—we had to move even though we had no money to do so. Maybe it had something to do with me being at the cusp of perimenopause with all the hormone fluctuations that go along with that, or that I've been dieting or that I became more lax about my diet after years of feeling okay even when I "cheat" a little. The bottom line is that all of a sudden I felt terrible again. At first I didn't connect it to my hypoglycemia, but after surfing the Internet and looking at a few hypo web sites, it became apparent that it was my hypoglycemia coming back with a vengeance.

Interestingly, I found that current advice for hypos was different than the advice I got from the dietitian about 15 years ago. Not only is table sugar bad for hypos, but so is honey, fruit juice concentrate and all sweeteners. And not only sweeteners are bad, but all refined carbs including all the white breads, white rice and white pasta that I've been eating. So is all the caffeine I was drinking. I found examples of the proper hypo diet on the Internet as well as several Internet-based support groups and bulletin boards.

When all this happened, in addition to dieting, I had been a vegetarian (an ovo-lacto vegetarian that only very rarely even had any fish). I found that even when I followed the hypo diet strictly, I didn't feel that well, not as well as I should have felt. Even on the hypo diet I had frequent sugar crashes, especially when I did a lot of exercise. Several other hypos I met on the Internet told me that I would have to go back to eating meat. I resisted for a long time and tried to just increase the amount of vegetarian protein I ate, but it didn't work. I started to keep a journal that not only recorded the food I was eating, but how I reacted to the food. It became apparent to me that, first of all, I had to stop dieting and pay more attention to my blood sugar than to losing weight. Once my blood sugar stabilized I could then try to lose weight again. Second of all, I did have to add some animal protein to my diet.

I did regain most of the weight that I had lost, but I felt a whole lot better. After my blood sugar had been stabilized for about a year or so, I started trying to lose weight again. It was hard finding a diet plan that worked without causing me to have hypo crashes. Last September I started on Weight Watchers' new Core program, which fit in very well with my hypo diet. I have lost nearly 35 lbs. on it so far without messing up my blood sugar balance, even when I exercise. I need to lose another 10-20 lbs. to get to my goal weight. Finally at 48 years old, I feel better than I remember ever feeling before.

Myra, a freelance writer and editor, lives in Monroe, NY.

Vitamins, minerals and herbs

In addition to diet and exercise, it is important to supplement with vitamins and minerals. I always thought that if I ate properly (and I assumed that I knew how to do this) I wouldn't need to take any "pills". Unfortunately, this isn't true, especially for hypoglycemics. Fluctuating blood sugar causes constant stress on the system and uses up vitamins and minerals much more quickly than normal.

The following sections list many of the vitamins, minerals and herbals that are useful for reducing hypoglycemia symptoms. Some of the supplements recommended also help to lessen the cravings for sugar and carbohydrates and some even appear to improve the underlying conditions that cause the hypoglycemia. The supplements are listed in alphabetical order with the most important supplements marked with an asterisk (*). At minimum, you should be taking a high quality multi-vitamin with minerals.

The first section lists thirty supplements that are suggested as useful for hypoglycemia in the literature. Please don't view this as a shopping list and fill your cart with 30 bottles of pills and powders. Instead, this section is intended to help you to have an informed conversation with your medical practitioner to decide which supplements may be right for you.

Interactions with medications you are already taking are a possibility even with well-tested supplements, so always talk to your doctor before adding anything other than the basic over-the-counter multi-vitamin and mineral preparations. No matter what supplements you decide to add, always check labels. Don't buy supplements that contain sugar and check for the inclusion of dairy, wheat or other fillers that could cause allergic reactions.

Be very careful when considering taking any product that does not indicate quantities—be sure to ask your doctor or nutritionist when this is the case. The label should show the botanical name of the plant, the part of the plant, the name and address of the manufacturer, a batch or lot number, the date of manufacturer, and the expiration date. Always be cautious when adding new drugs, vitamins or herbals to your diet.

The recommended daily allowances, or RDAs, are listed where available. Canada and the USA share nutrition research committees and have harmonized RDA numbers. When you see "RDA" before a dosage, that's the recommended daily allowance for both Canada and the USA. Where "RDA" doesn't appear, the dosage listed is taken from reputable nutrition catalogues. Dosages are listed with most of the supplements discussed, but in cases where RDAs haven't yet been determined dosages should be discussed with your health care provider.

*B Complex

If you take no other vitamins, you should at least take your B complex. The B complex improves digestion, and increases your body's ability to tolerate low glucose levels. They are often billed as "anti-stress" vitamins because of their beneficial effects on the brain and nervous system. They also help improve energy and are very useful in mitigating the symptoms of peri-menopause. Take your B complex plus extra amounts of the following B Vitamins. Remember to take them in the morning. They can affect your sleep if you take them just before bed.

*B1 – Thiamine

Thiamine is important for circulation, and assists in blood formation. It is needed for healthy growth and appetite and increases production of hydrochloric acid (HCL) needed for proper digestion. Vitamin B1 also helps with the health and proper function of your brain. Symptoms that you may not be getting enough B1 are mood swings or periodic depression. In severe cases, thiamine deficiency results in Beriberi, a disease of the nervous system.

Dosage and safety
RDA 1.5mg: Vitamin B1 can only be found naturally in whole, unprocessed foods, so many people are deficient in thiamine. Alcohol destroys B1, and even one drink a day can produce a deficiency in some people. Sugar, stress, tobacco, surgery and coffee also destroy thiamine.

*B2 – Riboflavin

Vitamin B2, also called riboflavin, is required for oxygen use. It helps lungs remove oxygen from the air and moves oxygen into the cells. It works in tandem with other B vitamins to metabolize fats, carbohydrates and proteins. Elderly people need more B2 and so do people who exercise a great deal. Alcoholics are often deficient in Vitamin B2.

Dosage and safety

RDA 1.7mg: Riboflavin is fragile and easily destroyed by processing and by light. Milk is an excellent source of riboflavin, but when it is sold in light permeable containers, most of the B2 is gone by the time you drink it. Keep in mind that tobacco, sugar, alcohol and coffee all inhibit absorption or use of Vitamin B2, and are all risk factors for a deficiency.

*B3 – Niacin / Niacinamide

Niacin seems to prevent abnormal drops in blood sugar and has been used with some success to treat alcoholism (alcoholics are often hypoglycemic). Vitamin B3 helps to convert fat to energy and is crucial in the production of the myelin sheath that protects the nerves. It is also needed for the production of insulin and the sex hormones. Niacin helps promote proper digestion by helping with the production of stomach acid and is used in the metabolism of carbohydrates.

Dosage and safety

RDA 20mg: B3 is easily absorbed, but not stored. Stress, some prescription drugs (antibiotics, for example) and alcohol and drug abuse all remove niacin from your body, so it is fairly easy to develop a deficiency. Sugar, tobacco, coffee, starch, corn and birth control pills also reduce the efficacy of niacin.

Niacin is very safe but should not be used if you have liver problems of any kind. It may cause flushing (reddened skin) due to the histamine it triggers, but histamine symptoms are not harmful and will disappear over time. Too much niacin may cause nausea and vomiting and it may elevate blood sugar in some diabetics. In this case, niacinamide can be used. It has the same benefits but has no effect on insulin production or use, so it may be preferred by hypoglycemics, too.

*B5 – Pantothenic Acid

Pantothenic acid is known as the stress vitamin because of its role in the manufacture of adrenal hormones. Many hypoglycemics have reduced adrenal function, so vitamin B5 is a very important addition to the hypoglycemic diet. Pantothenic acid is used in the metabolism of carbohydrates, fats, and glucose and supports the normal functioning of the gastrointestinal system.

Dosage and safety
RDA 5mg: Avoid coffee and alcohol—both reduce the effectiveness of Vitamin B5.

*B6 – Pyroxidine

Pyroxidine is involved in the manufacture of many of the proteins and hormones in your body and is needed for brain function. It is also used in making genetic material. Vitamin B6 is critical to your immune system and in antibody and red cell production. It aids digestion by helping metabolize fats, carbohydrates and proteins and through the production of digestive enzymes and HCL (stomach acid).

It has been used in the treatment of carpal tunnel syndrome with some success but more work is needed to determine the amount of improvement that can be expected without surgery.

Dosage and safety

RDA 2mg: Vitamin B6 enhances zinc absorption. Tobacco, coffee, alcohol and birth control pills all reduce the effectiveness of this important nutrient.

*B12 – Cyanocobalamin

Vitamin B12 is needed for proper growth and development of red blood cells. It is also helpful in ensuring proper digestion through the absorption of nutrition from foods and synthesis of protein.

A deficiency of B12 can result in pernicious anemia. Pernicious anemia was fatal until the 1920's when it was discovered that eating liver could reverse the disease. It was only later that it was discovered that liver was a good source of Vitamin B12.

Dosage and safety

RDA 6mcg: Meat is the only food source of Vitamin B12, so vegetarians must supplement their diet with this vitamin. Alcohol, tobacco, coffee and laxatives inhibit the absorption and action of B12, so habitual use of any of these should be avoided.

*Biotin

Biotin, part of the B Complex, is essential for cell growth, muscle tone and healthy skin and hair. Biotin also helps in the production of enzymes necessary for metabolism of sugars, fats and proteins. A deficiency of biotin results in a deficiency of glucose for energy. Supplementing with biotin can enhance your insulin sensitivity and improve the use of glucose in your liver. Vitamin B absorption depends on adequate biotin.

Dosage and safety

RDA 300mcg: Biotin has been tested for toxicity and there are no known toxic side effects even at large doses.

Brewer's Yeast

Brewer's yeast appears on many lists of supplements recommended for the treatment of hypoglycemia. One Danish study reported that people with hypoglycemia showed improvement in their symptoms after taking two tablespoons of brewer's yeast every day for one month.

Brewer's yeast contains chromium plus many B vitamins, amino acids and easily absorbable minerals. It contains all of the essential amino acids, fourteen minerals and seventeen vitamins plus zinc, iron, phosphorus and selenium. It is also a good source of protein and you can add it to soups and stews to increase their nutritional value. This is especially important if you are vegetarian because brewer's yeast includes many of the vitamins and nutrients that are generally found only in meat. Brewer's Yeast also aids in digestion because it encourages growth of good bacteria in your intestines.

Dosage and safety

Two tablespoons per day: Brewer's yeast is available in tablets, flakes or powder. Make sure you have brewer's yeast (used for making beer) and not baking yeast—it's not the same thing. Get your brewer's yeast from any good health food store.

Many sources caution against the use of brewer's yeast if

you have candidiasis (yeast overgrowth) or if you suffer frequent yeast infections, oral thrush or athlete's foot. New information suggests that brewer's yeast will not aggravate any of these conditions, but if you think it may be right for you, be sure to discuss it with your health care provider before taking it.

Don't use brewer's yeast if you have intestinal disease, you are allergic to yeast, or if your immune system is impaired. Don't exceed the daily dosage on the product label. It's alright to use brewer's yeast if you are pregnant, but whether pregnant or not, you may want to start with a small dosage, say one teaspoon or less per day, since brewer's yeast can cause bloating or gas until your system becomes used to it. You can work up slowly to one to two tablespoons of powder per day.

*Calcium

We all know that we need calcium to prevent osteoporosis and to build strong bones and teeth. But you can add glucose intolerance to the list of problems that could indicate a calcium deficiency. With magnesium, calcium helps in regulating blood sugar levels, and in metabolizing fats. Hypoglycemics often burn sugar rather than fat for energy, so calcium can help by improving fat metabolism. It's good for your digestion, too.

Other benefits of getting enough calcium are improved colon health, stress reduction, and faster healing (Calcium activates Vitamin K). Calcium is also needed for absorption of Vitamins A, C and B6.

You can increase your calcium intake by adding milk, molasses, nuts, dandelions, tofu, shellfish, eggs, wheat, collards or legumes to your diet.

Dosage and safety

RDA 1000mg: Remember to take your multivitamin—you need Vitamin D for proper absorption of calcium. Some of the drugs that block the absorption of calcium from your food are cortisone, aspirin, chemotherapeutic agents, and tetracyclines.

If you are diabetic, you should check with your doctor before supplementing with calcium, since some diabetics have been found to have too much calcium in their cells. Calcium can help with sleep, so try taking it before bed.

*Chromium

Chromium is the most important supplement for helping to improve hypoglycemia and insulin resistance in general. Numerous studies have shown that insulin just doesn't work without chromium, and there is evidence that chromium helps both hypoglycemics and diabetics. In addition, it may protect against stroke and heart attack by lowering elevated blood cholesterol and tryglyceride levels. It promotes weight loss because of improved fat burning, and helps convert fat to muscle.

You especially need chromium if you are diabetic, hypoglycemic or you eat a highly refined carbohydrate diet. Seniors, too, should supplement with chromium, since the body's absorption of nutrients isn't as effective as it is in young people. When you are down with the flu or cold, extra chromium may be necessary—blood chromium levels drop when you have a viral infection.

The crucial nature of chromium in animal health has been known since the 1950's, but human evidence only became available in the 1970's as doctors treated patients with intravenous nutrition. Some of these long-term patients developed high blood sugar levels even though they weren't diabetic. When chromium was added to the nutrition mix, these patients quickly improved, and their insulin injections were no longer necessary.

Studies have shown that simple sugars prompt chromium to be discharged in the urine—one source suggests that up to 20 percent more chromium leaves the body—so removing sugar from your diet is as important as adding chromium and both should be done together. Increasing your chromium may also decrease your sugar cravings, so supplementing with chromium may help you cut down your sugar consumption.

Chromium occurs naturally in organ meats, broccoli, mushrooms, whole grains, processed meats, peppers, milk, cheese, eggs and Brewer's Yeast. Most of us don't get even the 50mcg minimum from our diets, so supplementation would be a benefit, whether you are hypoglycemic or not. One source suggests that refinement of grains destroys most of the chromium, so even if you eat plenty of grains, you may not be getting as much chromium as you think.

Dosage and safety
RDA 200mcg: Make sure that you take chromium GTF

(Glucose Tolerance Factor), not chromium salts. Chromium picolinate is believed to be safe, but has come under question at the time of this writing. Chromium (in both picolinate and GTF forms) appears to be non-toxic even in high doses, but talk to your health care provider or your local pharmacist or health food storeowner. They should be able to tell you about the latest findings.

Some hypoglycemics have reported that they get maximum benefit by taking their chromium just before they eat.

*Magnesium

Magnesium is a crucial element for your heart, brain and kidneys. It is involved in thyroid production, and hormone, antibody and protein synthesis. Magnesium works with calcium for muscle contraction and helps produce energy, especially in muscle cells. Magnesium is also involved in producing stomach acid and digestive enzymes. It is especially important for hypoglycemics because it aids in the digestion of sugar, starches and fats and helps stabilize blood sugar levels. The secretion and action of insulin require magnesium.

Supplementing with magnesium is especially important if you are increasing your intake of refined carbohydrates or if you have too much calcium in your body (not uncommon in diabetics). Liver dysfunction is another reason you might want to supplement with magnesium. If you crave chocolate, it could be an indication that you are low in magnesium.

The dietary sources of magnesium include whole grains, nuts, seeds, cocoa, milk, green vegetables, seafood, brown rice, kidney and lima beans.

Dosage and safety

RDA 400mg: Don't exceed the recommended daily dosage. Too much or too little magnesium may cause depression. And don't take extra magnesium if you have kidney disease because it is the kidney that processes the magnesium.

*Manganese

Manganese is used in your body for fat and protein metabolism and the production of energy. It is needed for growth, maintenance of connective tissue, bone and cartilage and helps with fatty acid synthesis. Manganese is needed for the proper maintenance of blood glucose levels, so it is useful in treating diabetes and hypoglycemia. It is also useful in the treatment of epilepsy, anorexia and iron deficiency. The absorption of Vitamins C, B1 and E depend on sufficient amounts of manganese, so make sure your multivitamin supplement includes it.

Dietary sources of manganese include whole grain cereals, leafy vegetables, nuts and tea.

Dosage and safety

RDA 2-5mg: Take separate from calcium for best use by your body. Don't exceed the recommended dosage—high doses may cause hypertension and irreversible neurological disorders, and may interfere with absorption of other metals and minerals.

Selenium

Selenium is an essential trace mineral that helps enhance immunity by working in the production of antibodies. It is a free radical scavenger, so it helps to prevent oxidation that has been linked to premature ageing. Selenium is needed for proper operation of the thyroid gland and for protein synthesis in the liver. Selenium also appears to provide some protection from heart disease and can be used to cleanse the body of heavy metal poisoning.

Dietary sources of selenium include seafood, liver, kidney, whole grains, vegetables, garlic, Brazil nuts and walnuts, cottage cheese, oatmeal, chicken and turkey meat, enriched noodles and canned tuna. Brazil nuts have by far the largest concentration of selenium at 840mcg/oz. Most of the other sources contribute less than 100mcg per serving.

Selenium enters grains through the soil and there are parts of the world where the soil's reserve of selenium has been depleted through decades of over-use. If you live in those parts of North America, China and Russia where there is very little or no selenium in the soil, it is especially important that you ensure that the rest of your diet contains an adequate supply.

Dosage and safety
RDA 55mcg for adults: (60mcg for pregnant women, 70mcg if breast-feeding). Most people get enough selenium in their diets unless they live in a selenium-depleted area.

Too much selenium can result in a condition called selenosis, which produces symptoms of gastrointestinal upset, hair loss, white blotchy nails and mild nerve damage. One study suggests that a tolerable upper intake level for selenium is 400mcg/day.

*Vitamin C

Vitamin C is crucial for the production, development and strength of collagen needed for all connective tissue in your body. It is also important for the development and maintenance of healthy bones and teeth. Vitamin C strengthens the immune system and aids in healing. This important vitamin also increases the absorption of iron and protects against heavy metal toxicity. Most important for hypoglycemics, vitamin C supports the function of the adrenal glands and helps rebuild adrenals that are burned out—a condition common in hypoglycemics.

Citrus fruits like oranges and grapefruit are well-known sources of vitamin C, but today's grocery supply of citrus fruit may contain a lot less vitamin C than you think. Most of the citrus fruits we eat now are ripened in the back of a truck, rather than in the orchard, and it is the sun ripening that generates the vitamin C supply that we need.

Dosage and safety
RDA 60mg: This is the lower limit to prevent scurvy and many doctors are now recommending much larger doses. Vitamin C amounts up to 10 grams have been studied with no toxic effects discovered. It works best with magnesium and calcium and is inhibited by aspirin, antibiotics, tobacco, cortisone, fever and stress.

*Vitamin E

Vitamin E helps with circulation and energy and improves healing. It acts as an antioxidant for prevention of joint damage by free radicals. Vitamin E also neutralizes toxins and helps protect your eyes from too much sunlight.

Vitamin E is available in fruits, vegetables, grains and oils. Unfortunately, cooking and storage often destroy it so it is quite common to have a deficiency unless you take a supplement containing vitamin E.

Dosage and safety
RDA 10mg: Vitamin E has been found to be safe in dosages as high as 800mg/day and no toxicity has been noted even at much higher dosages than that.

*Zinc

Zinc is needed for proper release of insulin and many hypoglycemics may be deficient. Some of zinc's functions include cholesterol, protein and energy metabolism, growth, healing and immune function. Zinc is essential for protein synthesis and is needed for the transport of vitamin A. It is especially needed in pregnant women and childhood through to the end of adolescence. Elderly people often need more zinc because of decreased absorption and intake. Zinc supplementation may also be beneficial for patients with chronic diseases like diabetes.

Dietary sources include meat, eggs, seafood (oysters), milk, whole grains, spinach, soybeans and sunflower seeds. Keep in mind that zinc is destroyed when food is processed, so eat these foods in their natural form as often as possible.

Dosage and safety

RDA 15mg: Zinc absorption is reduced in the presence of alcohol, diuretics, cortisone, Tagamet and antacids. Stress causes zinc levels to drop rapidly. Too much zinc can cause impaired immune response, chronic nausea and vomiting and results in deficiencies of other minerals. Try to get your zinc from your diet and use a zinc supplement only under a doctor's care.

More supplements

The following list includes more supplements that are recommended for hypoglycemics. In most cases, there isn't much (or any) science to back up the claims of improvement of hypoglycemic symptoms. And if there is pretty good anecdotal evidence of benefit, the dosages and toxicity haven't really been tested. On the other hand, some promote general health by promoting good digestion. Good digestion is very important in metabolizing sugars properly. From that point of view, some of these, acidophilus, for example, may be a good addition to a hypoglycemia program.

With other supplements such as copper, the science is there, but proof of a specific benefit for hypoglycemia is not. If you think some of these sound good to you, discuss them with your doctor, or better yet, a holistic practitioner. Don't try this at home, folks!

Acidophilus

Acidophilus is a bacteria that helps digest protein, and helps promote the growth of the "good" bacteria that is always present in your digestive system. It is also one of the primary treatments for candidiasis (yeast overgrowth in the digestive system). Follow the instructions of your doctor or use the suggested dosage on the bottle. Remember, most acidophilus supplements must be stored in the refrigerator to maintain their effectiveness.

Carnitine

Carnitine behaves like an amino acid in that it converts stored body fat into energy. It increases the effectiveness of vitamin C and E and helps prevent fatigue. Important for heart health, carnitine prevents fat build-up in your heart, liver and muscles. Carnitine supplemental forms include *L-carnitine, DL-carnitine* and *acetyl-L-carnitine.* Check with your doctor and don't exceed the daily dose marked on the label.

Copper

Copper deficiency is not common, but is possible if you are using estrogen therapy or if you are suffering from post-partum depression. If you are taking mega-doses of vitamin C or supplementing with too much Zinc, you may need to supplement your copper intake, since large amounts of either of these can inhibit copper absorption. Copper imbalance is common in people prone to yeast infections. Having enough copper in your system will ensure that you are able to absorb and use iron. One of copper's most important functions is the protection of the myelin sheath that surrounds the nerves. If that's not enough, copper is also a natural anti-inflammatory and an anti-fungal agent.

Sources include liver, fish, soybeans, meats, seafood, nuts and seeds, whole grains and legumes, avocados, almonds, beets, broccoli, garlic, green leafy vegetables, lentils and lobster.

Dosage and safety

RDA 2mcg: Copper can be useful in treating hypoglycemia, but you should be tested before supplementing to be sure you have a deficiency. Never supplement with copper if you have Wilson's Disease.

Glucomannan

Glucomannan is a water-soluble dietary fiber derived from konjac root. It appears to have some effect in treatment of hypoglycemia caused by stomach surgery. This may be because it delays stomach emptying leading to a more gradual absorption of sugar.

Glucomannan is a bulk-forming laxative, so if you and your doctor feel that this fiber should be part of your treatment, start with a small dosage and build up slowly to reduce the possibility of gas and abdominal discomfort.

If you have a disorder of the esophagus, you should not take any fiber supplement in pill form since expansion in the esophagus could lead to obstruction. Preliminary studies suggest that some people may be sensitive to inhaled glucomannan powder. There are no well-known drug interactions with glucomannan.

Garlic

Garlic stimulates the immune system and is reputed to improve endurance and strength. It improves digestion, so it is also recommended in the treatment of candida overgrowth. For generations, garlic has been used for its natural antibiotic properties, and was used in the Second World War when penicillin ran low. It is also a natural anti-fungal and is reputed to lower cholesterol.

While some sources claim that garlic relieves low blood sugar, other sources say it *lowers* blood sugar and recommend it for diabetics because it increases insulin. Don't try it except on the advice of your doctor—there just hasn't been enough testing. No side effects have been noted (except, of course, vampire repulsion!)

Glutamine

Glutamine is an amino acid that appears naturally in the body in great quantities. It is actively transported or used in almost all of the tissues of the body and is highly concentrated in the brain. Glutamine supports pancreatic growth and function and helps your body to better absorb the nutrients from the food you eat. Glutamine stimulates the immune system and is useful in recovery from illness—glutamine depletion can be dramatic when you are ill or injured.

Of special interest to hypoglycemics, glutamine suppresses insulin when the blood sugar is low and stimulates sugar release from the cells to help bring the blood sugar levels back to normal. In addition, it has been known to help suppress sugar and alcohol cravings.

Effective use of glutamine requires vitamin B6 and manganese, and glutamine is needed for efficient use of vitamin B3. Dietary sources of glutamine include pork, poultry, eggs and dairy products, wheat germ, oats and avocados.

Don't supplement glutamine if you are prone to mania, and even if you aren't, you'll sleep better if you don't take it after three p.m. For best effect, take between meals and with pyridoxal-5-phosphate. Don't ever take more than the recommended dosage, since over-dosing can result in a reversal of the effect. Studies have not shown toxicity, but you shouldn't take glutamine if you suffer from acute liver or kidney failure.

Glutathione

Glutathione is an amino acid that inhibits formation of free radicals. It aids in red blood cell integrity, protects immune cells and may even increase T-cells. It is needed for the breakdown of glucose and helps regulate blood sugar.

Hydrochloric Acid

Hydrochloric acid, or HCL, is part of the essential stomach acid required for proper digestion. Overgrowth of candida results in an alkaline digestive system, so HCL supplementation is considered especially useful in candidiasis. Adequate HCL is required for use of B vitamins and minerals and supplementation may be required if you are a senior since HCL production decreases with age.

Don't use HCL if you have an ulcer.

Quercetin

Because quercetin is a natural antihistamine, it is useful in reducing the effects of allergies. It is also anti-inflammatory and helps increase immunity. Dietary sources include apple skins, dark berries such as blueberries, blackberries and dark cherries; also citrus fruits, onions, parsley, tea, and red wine. Since alcohol is off the list for hypoglycemics, stick to the fruit and (decaffeinated) tea.

Quercetin works best when used with bromelain, an enzyme found in pineapple, and when used together the amount of bromelain should be equal to the amount of quercetin.

No side effects have been reported, but because of the possibility of interaction with other drugs, you should be sure to talk to your health care provider before adding quercetin to your dietary regimen.

Spirulina

Spirulina is a blue green algae used to treat fatigue and excessive appetite. This plant certainly deserves a closer look because it is reputed to contain 71 percent digestible protein. This would make it a great addition to a hypoglycemic or vegetarian diet.

It comes in capsules and powder—check with your health store staff and holistic doctor to see if spirulina might be right for you.

Supplements to use with extra care

The following supplements appear in the supplement listings, but there is little or no scientific backing for most of the claims made. Please talk to your health care provider before trying any of these.

Aloe Vera

According to some sources aloe vera helps with stress by boosting the immune system and promotes good colon bacteria. One source lists aloe vera as "Very Important" for the treatment of hypoglycemia, but no backup studies or standard dosages are listed. Use this one with care and only under the supervision of your doctor.

Juniper berries

According to some sources, juniper berries help to strengthen the kidneys and adrenal glands, and assist in preventing hypoglycemia. They have been used for years in folk medicine, so small amounts probably aren't harmful but there isn't any science to suggest that there would be particular benefits for hypoglycemics. Many supplements and teas sold on the internet contain juniper berries, but it is hard to say whether or not there are standards for their quality or purity. Best to avoid them unless your health practitioner particularly suggests them.

Licorice root

Licorice root is listed in the literature as a supplement that helps strengthen the adrenal glands and regulate blood sugar. It is reputed to be able to raise blood sugar without a corresponding insulin reaction.

Licorice root has not been rigorously tested, so I do not recommend its use. If you feel that it might help you, be sure to use it for no more than seven days at a time. Do not use licorice root at all if you have high blood pressure or if you are retaining water.

Ginseng

Ginseng is highly touted for its ability to improve stress handling, rebuild adrenal glands, aid digestion and increase mental clarity and accuracy (not proven).

It has also been reported to help regulate blood sugar levels, but some reports say it *causes* hypoglycemia. There is sugar in ginseng, and perhaps that explains why it might cause hypoglycemia in some people.

American ginseng is less potent and perhaps safer than Siberian ginseng, but no ginseng should be taken if you are obese, suffer from high blood pressure or any heart disorder. You should also avoid ginseng during acute illness or infection or when constipated, or if you have schizophrenia or breast cancer. Because of hormonal effects, you should not take ginseng if you are pregnant or breastfeeding—some sources say that Siberian ginseng should be avoided by anyone under forty for the same reason.

Use of ginseng should be on a regimen of no more than three weeks on; two weeks off. Possible side effects include diarrhea, sleep disturbance, headache, hypertension, skin rash, a decreased diuretic effect and increased bleeding in menopausal women. There are also interactions with the following drugs: warfarin, insulin, phenelzine, caffeine, digitalis, guarana and hormone therapy.

Since it is often mislabeled and can contain impurities, it would be my recommendation not to use it at all unless it is part of your health-care provider's treatment program and she is aware of your medical history and all of your other medications. That being said, ginseng is present in small amounts in some reputable supplements.

Herbs and supplements to avoid

Here are some herbs that you will see in the literature in the context of regulating blood sugar. Read all of the information carefully, since some are suitable only for diabetics because they *decrease* blood sugar. I would recommend staying away from all of the herbs mentioned on this list.

Bitter Melon

Never use bitter melon—it lowers blood sugar, and is sometimes used by diabetics.

Gymnema sylvestre/Gymnema extract

Gymnema sylvestre is used to normalize blood glucose function by repairing, revitalizing and regenerating the beta cells of the pancreas. It should **never** be used by hypoglycemics, since it *INCREASES* insulin.

Kombucha tea

Kombucha tea appears frequently enough in the herb listings that I felt I should mention it here, but it has not been sufficiently tested for effectiveness and safety. Side effects include nausea and vomiting and toxicity testing has not been done. Some reports even say that kombucha tea can *cause* hypoglycemia, possibly because it contains caffeine.

Now that your brain is full of vitamins and minerals (or at least their names) let's get into the nitty-gritty of the hypoglycemia diet.

Chapter 7

What can I eat?

■■■■**Ann's Story**

I am a reactive hypoglycemic. According to the literature that means I react negatively to sugar and simple starches, usually two to four hours after eating these foods. In fact, I will react to these foods in 15–30 minutes, responding with flushing extending through the face and torso, feelings of extreme fatigue and weakness, faintness and sleepiness. If I get a particularly bad response, I often have to lie down and will sleep for 30–60 minutes. I get this response when I either wait too long to eat or eat foods that I shouldn't. Once after eating a roasted marshmallow while camping, I experienced a reaction similar to being drunk (I could not talk properly and I could not walk straight). Sometimes when I am particularly hungry I will get disoriented, be unable to talk properly, and if walking, will tend to lean to the right as I walk, again similar to being drunk. I appear to be particularly reactive and my blood sugar will plummet if I am not very careful.

I was diagnosed as a reactive hypoglycemic 12 years ago after two blood glucose tests. The first showed nothing, the second showed reactive hypoglycemia. I realize, looking back, that I have probably been hypoglycemic all my life, but it has gotten progressively worse, first in my early twenties when I started to faint mid-morning if I didn't eat and when I was particularly active. Then it became severe during pregnancy and after my daughter was born.

After the birth of my daughter, I rapidly lost weight, losing my pregnancy weight in the first month and going on to lose an additional twenty-five lbs. Since I was slim to begin with and quite petite, I began to look positively anorexic going down to a size one. The doctor thought I might be suffering from "post-partum blues" as I was having anxiety attacks and felt quite depressed. I was unable to continue nursing after six months as I ran out of milk, and I couldn't seem to gain weight no matter what I ate. Sometimes I'd feel worse after eating then I did before, feeling faint, weak (like I had no muscles in my body) and incredibly tired. I saw a nutritionist who recommended that I try eating frequently and suggested that I get a test for hypoglycemia. The result of this test was normal.

I didn't get better so I asked to have the test again. This test showed that I was a reactive hypoglycemic. Now I had a diagnosis, but I really didn't have much else. The endocrinologist told me to eat like a diabetic. It helped somewhat, but not a lot.

So began over a decade of discovery, and I don't feel that I've found all the answers yet. I went to the library, bookstores and websites in search of information. I'd find a tidbit here and a tidbit there. I saw a naturopath who recommended I try "The Zone" diet that cuts a lot of carbohydrates out of the diet. This didn't work. I also tried "Sugar Busters", and high protein diets. None of them made a lot of difference. The diet that finally made a difference to my life was the Glycemic Diet based on the glycemic index. The glycemic index ranks carbohydrates by the effect they have on blood sugar levels. Glucose has a ranking of 100. The higher the number, the higher the gylcemic response. Eating the low-glycemic way has made a significant difference in helping me balance my blood sugars. This diet consists of ensuring that you have protein and a low glycemic carbohydrate (usually fruit and vegetables) at every meal and at least two, preferably three snacks a day. It also includes having fat at each meal (the good kind such as olive oil).

My diet now consists of:

■ Breakfast: (protein and fruit) Usually frozen or fresh berries or protein and granola (no wheat, no added honey or sugar, just whole grains). My protein often consists of cottage cheese. Note, yogurt doesn't have enough protein to be useful. Eggs are also good.

■ Snack: Usually soy nuts (other nuts are good as well but I am allergic to nuts), low fat cheese and an apple or other fruit, or cottage cheese and berries (frozen or fresh)

■ Lunch: Two or three types of vegetables or a robust salad (e.g., not iceberg lettuce), protein such as a chicken breast, fat in the form of olive oil, or a handful of olives. Fish and seafood make good protein as well, but I am allergic to them. Sometimes I have soy instead of chicken. I always have fruit for dessert.

■ Dinner is very similar to lunch, but my family likes a variety of meats so we may have pork chops/roast, or ground beef or a steak. Again, I have lots of vegetables. My family likes a potato, rice or pasta. I eat as little of this as possible or none at all.

Guidelines that have worked for me:

■ No more than one grain a day, usually breakfast with the granola or maybe a slice of multi-grain toast. Note: frequently commercial multigrain bread is full of sugar (glucose, caramel, raisin puree) and can have a high glycemic response.

■ Eat nothing that is white (potato, rice, bread, etc.)

■ Watch for hidden sugars in food (glucose, fructose, corn syrup, dextrose, etc.)

111

- *Avoid anything "lite" (e.g., salad dressings). Manufacturers tend to replace fat with sugar*
- *Eat as many vegetables at a meal as I can (2 to 3)*
- *Eat as many foods in their natural state as possible (e.g., avoid fast food, pre-prepared meals)*
- *Eat whole fruit, particularly berries*
- *Eat a mixture of protein, low glycemic carbohydrates (e.g., vegetables), and a good fat (e.g., olive oil, olives, avocado) at every meal*
- *Eat protein and a low glycemic carbohydrate for every snack (usually 3 per day)*
- *Eat every 2 to 3 hours and have a snack right before going to bed*
- *Always carry food with me (e.g., cheese sticks, soy nuts, dried apples)*
- *Get enough sleep (at least 7 hours)*
- *Exercise*

Eating and living this way has not been easy. I have a small, but successful business with clients around the world. I travel 30+ weeks of the year for 3 to 5 days of the week and I teach a course at the university. A slow week for me is usually 65 hours long. I'm married with one child. I also have two ageing parents and I try to make time for my family when I can. Compounding my hypoglycemia is asthma and food allergies (I'm allergic to a lot of protein sources like fish, nuts, seafood, lentils, many legumes and some other vegetables).

I'm not always "good" about sticking to my diet and getting enough sleep and exercise is very difficult. I sometimes fall "off the wagon" and succumb to potato chips or popcorn as a snack, but I feel the results the next day. If I don't get enough sleep, I end up having problems with my blood sugar for weeks afterwards. I occasionally allow myself a small piece of 70 percent chocolate. I need to eat again within half an hour, but sometimes it is worth it.

My diet was already restricted before and it is even more so now. Sometimes I am very frustrated and wish I could be "normal" like other people or just take a pill. However, considering the diseases that many people have, I realize I am fortunate that my disease can be managed with diet, and most importantly I have no choice but to eat and live the life that many doctors are advocating as the healthiest way to live. I may have asthma and hypoglycemia, but I'm a healthy "sick person".

Ann Rockley is an author and (very busy!) business person living in Toronto, Canada.

What are we eating?

Books, web sites, newspapers and television shows about diets and dieting abound. If you were to ask, "Do we really need another diet?" you would be asking a legitimate question. We already have "Eat Right for Your Type", "Dr. Kushner's Personality Type Diet", "The Zone" diet, and dozens of others.

I would argue that each of us needs just one more diet, our own.

Many of us, and hypoglycemics especially, are sensitive to particular foods. Over time, we need to work out which foods make us feel good and which foods don't. Keeping a record of how we respond to various foods is the first step in learning to eat what we need.

There was a time when I would have been very skeptical of the previous statements. For one thing, I always fight any implication that I might not be "normal" (whatever that means). For another, I always thought, "If it was good enough for my grandparents, it should be good enough for me."

That sounds great, except that we are not eating the same foods or the same quality of foods that our grandparents ate. When I imagine my grandparents on the farm on the prairies, I know that sugar was hard to come by and the occasional hard candy was a major treat. And even though the basis of their diet was similar—many of us still eat a diet based on "meat and potatoes"—the quality and quantity of the foods have changed significantly. Even the bread, still a staple, has changed. We now refine all of the nutrients out of the flour, so the bread just doesn't pack the same punch. Here are some examples of the changes that have taken place over the last 100 years.

Almost all of the food eaten on the farm of one hundred years ago was home grown. For most families, sugar had to be purchased, so it was used sparingly. All of the vegetables were organically grown—no chemicals were available for weed or pest control, so none were used. The flour was less refined (the grinding technology wasn't what it is today!) so the flour was actually less stripped of goodness than it is now. The soil had not yet been overused, so vitamins and minerals (selenium, for example) from the soil enriched everything that was grown.

Now, almost all of the fruits and vegetables we eat are grown with the benefits of pesticides and herbicides and high-tech fertilizers. Even if you buy organically grown produce today, it will still not have the same nutrient content as the fruits and vegetables we would have eaten one hundred years ago. We now have access to a much wider selection of fruits and vegetables, and many more are available fresh all year round. This may lessen the effect of the reduced nutritive value of the vegetables and fruits we eat, but shipping and storage also causes loss of nutrients. Any way you slice it, we just don't have the quality we used to.

Much of the food was home prepared and preserved. The fruit and vegetables were fresh and contained no preservatives or artificial ingredients (and now we pay extra for organic). Sugar wasn't always available, and farm wives wouldn't often have had time to make elaborate desserts. Sweets were a rarity for many families, saved for special occasions.

With the affluence of most segments of our society growing so quickly, our society's taste for sugar and sweet things has grown over the past one hundred years. Our cravings for sweets and empty carbohydrates have led us down the garden path from obesity and diabetes straight through to hypoglycemia and Syndrome X.

Highly processed packaged foods are another of the dubious improvements of the 20th century and it can be difficult to understand just what we are eating. It's time to get smart about what we buy and consume.

Read labels

Whether or not we are hypoglycemic, we need to start reading labels. We need to understand what we are putting into our bodies. The food we eat provides the fuel for everything we do, and just like our cars, good fuel makes for a better ride. We understand that buying unleaded fuel of the proper octane level keeps our cars running at optimum performance. Our bodies are no different, except that, unlike our cars, we cannot replace them when they wear out.

In addition to finding out what the ingredients are, by reading the labels we can also find out (approximately) how much of each ingredient there might be. The ingredients are listed in order by the amount in which they appear in the list. The food product contains more of the top ingredient than the second one, and more of the third ingredient than the one that appears fourth on the list.

Here's a sample ingredients list from a can of brand name chicken corn chowder:

chicken broth
potatoes
seasoned chicken
corn
water
carrots
canola or soybean oil
celery
modified corn starch
cream
enriched wheat flour
butter
bacon
yeast extract and hydrolyzed wheat gluten
chicken fat
dehydrated onions
sugar
potato starch
salt
soy protein isolate
spice
beta carotene

In addition to finding out that, yes, there is sugar in this soup; we can also deduce that it is a very small amount, since it appears way down the list. Vegetarians already know that this soup is not for them—it contains chicken and bacon. Celiacs and wheat-sensitive people will also avoid this soup because of the added gluten and wheat. The main ingredients are potatoes, chicken and corn, and, of course, chicken broth. These would still be the top ingredients if you had made this soup yourself, so this is probably a pretty good product. As an added bonus, the list doesn't include anything I can't pronounce—a good sign! Having said that this is a pretty good product, it should be said that many hypoglycemics still would not be able to eat this soup. Many cannot tolerate even the smallest amounts of sugar. In addition, high carbohydrate meals like this soup (mostly potatoes and corn) are generally not well tolerated by hypoglycemics.

Compare the soup ingredients to the list on a box of name brand low fat crackers:

enriched flour

vegetable oil shortening

dehydrated vegetable and seasoning blend (carrot, onion, celery, cabbage, tomato, red bell pepper—all treated with sulphites, dextrose, salt, wheat starch, monosodium glutamate, wheat flour, spices and seasoning, sugar, hydrolyzed plant protein, colour, disodium inosinate, disodium guanylate)

sugar

salt

ammonium bicarbonate

glucose-fructose or invert liquid sugar

monocalcium phosphate,

sodium bicarbonate

hydrolyzed plant protein

protease

This list is much more daunting, and not at all like something I would make at home. Do we really want to eat something that contains chemicals you we can hardly pronounce? These crackers also contain a significant amount of sugar. First, all the vegetables are coated in a sugar mixture and then the cracker itself also contains sugar.

Are we really meant to eat this way? The two products I've listed really aren't that bad when compared to the many kinds of bad "food" available in grocery stores. But this is representative of the way many of us eat today.

It is clear to all of us by now that there are "foods" that no one should be eating.

"Fat-free", "Low fat" and "Sugar-free" foods

Be very suspicious of "fat-free", "low fat" and "sugar-free" foods.

I used to think I was being really "good" buying ultra-low fat mayonnaise. When I started to really look at the labels, though, I noticed that the ultra-low fat version had more sugar added than the low fat version and that low fat mayonnaise has more sugar than the regular mayonnaise. This was not the exception but the rule. And in addition to adding more sugar, in many cases, the lower fat versions of foods also contained more chemical additives. Low fat and ultra-low fat may sound like good ideas at first, but stay away from them.

"Sugar-free" is another problem. "Sugar-free" never means "sweetener-free"—it invariably means that some other sweetener was used. Best case, it will be something like white grape juice, but usually it is an artificial sweetener like aspartame. Some artificial sweeteners raise blood sugar almost as much as "real" sweeteners, and besides, they are chemicals whose long-term effects on our bodies are not really known. Hypoglycemic or not, it is best to avoid all of them.

119

Testing foods to see what works for you

Now that we know how great an effect what we eat has on our well being, it's time to really start paying attention to how we feel when we eat different foods. Our bodies are trying to tell us what they need—it's time to start listening.

Most of us already have some rules about food. For instance, Joe says, "I never eat peanuts. They upset my stomach." Or Susan may say, "I don't like to eat chili or baked beans because of the gas". Most of us have foods we don't like to eat because they "don't agree with us". Perhaps you don't drink coffee in the evening because it affects your sleep.

Having hypoglycemia means that we need to take the next step. Hypoglycemics are often very sensitive to the blood-sugar-raising effects of various foods. As an example, I used to drink fruit drinks, not often, but for a change now and then. When I first started to keep track of how foods made me feel, I realized that within ten minutes of drinking the fruit drink, I had a bad headache. At the time, I was having headaches almost every day, so I hadn't noticed that fruit drinks were one of the causes.

Some foods may make you feel sleepy, or twitchy, or or as with any juice and me, give you a headache. Some may make you feel spacey and dilate your pupils. It's not uncommon for hypoglycemics to react this way to pasta or other high-carbohydrate meals.

In addition to feeling better and reducing or eliminating unpleasant food-related symptoms, tracking what you eat may also uncover food allergies. The best way I know of to adjust your diet for your own well-being is to keep a food journal.

Keeping a food journal

Start by tracking everything you eat for a few days. Write down the time of day, what you eat and how much, and how it makes you feel. Do you feel satisfied or do you still feel hungry? Do you feel light-headed or sleepy? How about an hour or two hours after? Are you hungry again or do you feel sick?

Keeping track at this level of detail can be time consuming at first, but it is worthwhile because you'll begin to make the link between what you eat and drink and the symptoms you experience. You may not need to keep track for more than a few days to learn a great deal.

See table 1 for the chart I used to track my eating when I first started taking charge of my hypoglycemia.

Before the journal, I tried to ignore how I felt as much as possible. I was too busy to feel crummy, so I just pretended I was fine. I remember being shocked one day when my daughter watched me take a pain killer and said "You always have a headache". I realized that she was right—I was taking painkillers every day. I had no idea what to do about it, so I ignored it and kept taking the painkillers.

A friend of mine told me about the food journal idea. I put it off for months because it sounded so time consuming. When I did begin, I started grudgingly. The first day or two were difficult, but after that I found that I was starting to

Table 1: Sample Food Journal

Date	Time	Food/Amount	How do I feel?
Today	7:00am	Bagel & cream cheese	8:30 stuffed; a little spacey
			9:00 shaky; hungry again
	9:00am	Apple	Much better
	10:00	hungry again 10 almonds	Feel better
	12:00	Lunch: ham sandwich with mustard on whole wheat bread; milk	Fine
	12:30	8 oz apple juice	12:40 sudden headache (don't want to do that again!)
	1:00 pm	Celery and cheese	Hungry again
	1:30		Feel great
	3:00	Salad with meat and cheese	
	6:00	Supper: Salad, 3 oz. grilled fish	Not hungry till supper, must have been a good snack!
	9:00	6 rice crackers with almond butter	Hungry, need a snack before bed

think ahead. I started to take note of how I felt all the time and I began to link how I was feeling to what I had eaten.

Starting the journal forced me to pay attention, but best of all, I could begin to figure out what to do about how I was feeling.

To start your food journal, copy Table 1 and carry it with you. Start journalling with the first thing you put into your mouth in the morning, and pay close attention to how you feel. Ask yourself these questions:

■ If you were hungry before you ate, did you stop being hungry after you ate?

■ How soon were you hungry again?

■ Did you feel especially energized after you ate?

■ Were you tired after you ate?

■ Did you have a headache or muscle aches that appeared or got worse after you ate?

Write your answers in the food journal. If you notice an effect that you think might be caused by a food, wait a few days and try the food again. Try to have it on its own, without any other foods just before or after it, and take note of how you feel. If you have the same reaction to the food again, you could have an allergy or sensitivity to that particular food. This will alert you so that you can begin to limit or eliminate foods that cause you discomfort. Keep in mind that the symptoms of some food sensitivities take several days to show up, making it difficult to see a link to a particular food. I only found out about my wheat sensitivity, for example, after avoiding wheat for a couple of weeks and finding that my eczema had disappeared.

123

If you still have sugar in your diet, keeping a food journal will give you a clearer sense of just how much sugar bothers you. I have been recommending cutting it out completely and many hypoglycemics do. If you are still struggling with that, your food journal will show you just how important a role sugar plays in how you feel. Once you link sugar with feeling "bad" it will be easier to cut it out of your diet.

After a couple of weeks, cut out those foods that you have found cause unpleasant side effects. You may find that you feel a lot better quite quickly. Stick to these dietary changes for a few weeks and *congratulate yourself!* You are taking charge of your own health and feeling better through your own actions. That feeling of control is wonderful and it will help motivate you for everything from finally starting that special project to taking the next step in improving your diet.

As you refine your diet, you may want to use the food journal to work out what your carbohydrate to protein ratio should be. For most people, this doesn't have to be exact or complicated. For this step, use the journal to find out which leaves you feeling better, steak and potatoes or steak and a salad. If you are able to eat pasta (whole grain is best), are you more comfortable after spaghetti and meatballs or spaghetti with a vegetable dish? These experiments will help to show you how much carbohydrate you can tolerate. I found that pasta doesn't work well for me, even when it is whole grain, so when I eat it occasionally, I limit it to half a cup and always have protein with it (meat sauce or cheese or both).

As you work on this stage, spend some time experimenting with breakfast. You don't have to have "breakfast food" for breakfast. Eat whatever gives you that boost you need to get your day going. As an example, I found that I felt more satisfied with whole grain toast and almond butter than I did with oatmeal and an egg. I have heard lots of very interesting breakfast menus (like tuna salad), and there are no wrong answers—eat what works for you.

Some people I know of have an ounce or two of steak for breakfast. Others eat lentils (they are high in protein, too). Nothing is too weird if it helps you get through your day feeling healthy and clear-headed.

Keep in mind that this is a process. Once you figure out what foods you shouldn't be eating, you'll start to work on foods to replace them with. This takes practice and it could take quite a while to work out some new menus. Use the workbook at the end of the book to help you make your diet changes.

Will this take an effort? Certainly. Will it be worth it? Absolutely! Having your body working better than ever will make it all worthwhile.

What the experts say...

There are many dietary approaches to managing your hypoglycemia and I'll introduce you to a few in the next sections. Many are not strictly aimed at hypoglycemics, but are followed by many hypoglycemia sufferers. I'll tell you about them and the good and bad points. Most of them will work well for hypoglycemics with some modifications.

Glycemic index

Dr. David Jenkins developed the glycemic index at the University of Toronto in Canada while researching diet for diabetics and first published his findings in 1981. The glycemic index (GI) is a ranking of foods on a scale from zero to 100 according to how much the blood sugar levels rise after eating them. A low GI number means that the food has a small effect on blood sugar, while a large number means that the food has a greater effect on blood sugar.

The glycemic index is still controversial, and, in fact, the two major groups studying the glycemic index (University of Sydney, Australia and The Glycemic Research Institute in Washington, DC) disagree on many points, including how it should be represented. (The Glycemic Research Institute lists foods simply as "acceptable" or "unacceptable" while the Australia group gives each food a number). Although you would think that information about the blood sugar effects of foods would be of special importance and interest to diabetics, as of March 2002, the American Diabetes Association still hadn't accepted the GI as having value for their membership. To be fair, though, the ADA was funding a study of the glycemic index as recently as 2004. The Canadian Diabetes Association does endorse use of the GI by diabetics in planning their food choices.

Professor Jennie Brand-Miller and her team at the School of Molecular and Microbial Biosciences at the University in Sydney have made great strides in understanding how different foods affect blood sugar and have measured the glycemic indices for many new foods. A large list has already been compiled, and you will be able to find it on the internet (check the sources at the end of the book).

The table below (see Table 2) shows the GI's for a few different foods. This sampling uses a base food of glucose and assigns it the number 100. All other foods are ranked above and below 100 based on how eating them affects the blood sugar response. There is another glycemic index that uses white bread as the base food. White bread is assigned the value 100, and all other foods are compared to it. This is why you will sometimes see different index values for the same foods.

Testing the glycemic index of a new food is costly and time consuming because human volunteers are used. Each volunteer eats a portion of the food being tested and then has their blood tested at intervals after that. The size of the portion is that amount of the food containing 50 grams of carbohydrate. Not all foods are included on the lists, and not only because researchers haven't yet tested them. Foods composed primarily of proteins or fats are not included because it was found that these foods have only a very small effect on blood sugar. Other foods that are missing include foods for which it is just too difficult to eat enough to get 50 grams of carbohydrate. Just imagine how much celery you would have to eat to get 50 grams of carbohydrate!

Many factors also affect the glycemic index of foods, including:

▌ *Amount of cooking:* The glycemic index of potatoes and pasta increase when they are cooked, and in the case of pasta, cooking past the al dente point raises the GI even more. The GI of brown rice, on the other hand, doesn't change much when it is cooked.

127

Table 2: Glucose-based index showing how to improve your food choices.

High GI Food	GI	Try substituting with...	GI
Bagel, 1 small, plain 2.3 oz.	72	Apple, 1 medium, 5 oz.	38
Basmati white rice, boiled, 1 cup, 6 oz.	58	Uncle Ben's Converted rice, 1 cup, 6 oz.	44
French baguette, 1 oz.	95	Taco shells, 2 shells, 1 oz.	68
White bread, 1 slice, 1 oz	70	Pumpernickel, whole grain, 1 slice, 1 oz.	51
Bread stuffing from mix, 2 oz.	74	Baked beans, ½ cup, 4 oz.	48
Rice Krispies, Kelloggs, 1 ½ cups	82	All-Bran with extra fiber, Kellogg's, ½ cup, 1 oz	51
Vanilla wafers, 7 cookies, 1 oz.	77	Oatmeal cookie, 1, ⅔ oz.	55
Ice cream, 10% fat, vanilla, ½ cup, 2.2 oz.	61	Yogurt, nonfat, fruit flavored, with sugar, 8 oz.	33
Linguini, thin, cooked, 1 cup, 6 oz.	55	Fettuccine, cooked, 1 cup, 6 oz.	32
Banana, 1 medium, 5 oz.	55	Pear, fresh, 1 medium, 5 oz.	38
Kidney beans, red, canned & drained, ½ cup, 4.3 oz.	52	Kidney beans, red, boiled, ½ cup, 3 oz.	27
Macaroni and Cheese Dinner, Kraft, 1 cup, 7 oz.	64	Macaroni, cooked 1 cup, 6 oz.	45
Milk, skim, 1 cup, 8 oz.	32	Milk, whole, 1 cup, 8 oz.	27
Oat bran muffin, 1, 2 oz.	60	Apple cinnamon muffin, 1, 2 oz.	44
Gatorade, 1 cup, 8 oz.	78	Orange juice, 1 cup, 8 oz.	46
Pizza, cheese & tomato, 2 slices, 8 oz.	60	Ravioli, meat-filled, cooked, 1 cup, 9 oz.	39
Potatoes, red-skinned, baked, 1 medium, 4 oz.	93	Sweet potato, peeled, boiled, ½ cup mashed, 3 oz.	54
French fries, 4.3 oz.	75	Power Bar, Performance, chocolate, 1 bar	58
Pretzels, 1 oz	83	Peanuts, roasted, salted, ½ cup, 2.5 oz.	14

Source: GI numbers for the various foods are taken from *The Glucose Revolution* by Jennie Brand-Miller, Ph.D., Thomas M.S. Wolever, M.D., Ph.D., Stephen Colagiuri, M.D., Kaye Foster-Powell, M. Nutr. & Diet.

▌ *Amount of processing:* Most processing removes fiber and fiber slows the blood response. Whole oats have a lower GI than oatmeal, because the processing needed to make oatmeal has already begun to break down the fiber.

▌ *Amount of fat and protein:* Fat and protein both slow the glycemic response, and adding fat and protein when you eat carbohydrates improves your chances of avoiding a sugar spike. Don't take this as permission, however, to load on the butter! You should still be avoiding the "bad" fats.

The concept of **Glycemic Load** was developed in response to concerns that large amounts of low glycemic foods might still cause unacceptable increases in the blood sugar level. The glycemic load (GL) links serving size to the glycemic index so that it is easier to use. Carrots, for example, have a very high glycemic index (higher than white bread), but this was measured with 50 grams of carbohydrate. Since one carrot has only about 4 grams of carbohydrate, you would have to eat a lot of carrots to get a huge blood sugar response.

On the other hand, pasta has a lower glycemic index, but a serving of pasta contains about forty grams of carbohydrate. This means that the blood sugar response you will have with a plate of pasta will be several times higher than even a whole serving of carrots.

Since low blood sugar is often caused by excess insulin that our bodies produce after eating, it makes sense to eat foods that cause a smaller increase in blood sugar so that we trigger a smaller insulin response. With this in mind, it makes sense to choose foods from the lower end of the glycemic index as much as possible. Many sources suggest choosing foods that have glycemic indices (GI's) of 50 or less. It may sound like just one more limit, one more rule to follow, but think of it as just one more way to compare foods and make food choices.

Low fiber carbohydrates are associated with the highest GI numbers. A cake donut, for instance, has a GI value of 76, and this is without icing. This is another way of proving what we already knew. Donuts cause a large increase in blood sugar, paving the way for a big sugar crash, so they are a very poor choice for hypoglycemics.

The glycemic index is full of surprises, too. Most of us eat lots of rice and potatoes. Almost all types of rice and potatoes have GI's of over 50. There are even types of rice that have GI's of over 100.

You will also notice that many whole grains fall on the bottom half of the index, that is, under 50, while many refined grains have GI's of over 50. In Chapter 4, we learned that hypoglycemia can be followed by insulin resistance and, eventually, diabetes. So it stands to reason that a diet of low glycemic foods including whole grains may even help prevent diabetes.

Given the difficulty of maintaining a stable blood sugar level, any tools we can use to help us figure it out are welcome. The glycemic index is one such tool.

The glycemic index is great, as far as it goes. But it is not a diet, and has nothing to say about what you should and shouldn't eat. It doesn't say "Don't eat sugar" or "Don't eat white bread". It simply tells you what your body's sugar response is likely to be when you choose certain foods.

Dr. Brand-Miller has written a diet book (*The Glucose Revolution* by Jennie Brand-Miller, Ph.D., Thomas M.S. Wolever, M.D., Ph.D., Stephen Colagiuri, M.D., Kaye Foster-Powell, M. Nutr. & Diet.) based on the Glycemic index. She describes the standard low-fat, high-carbohydrate diet, with the difference that she recommends basing most meals on low GI foods. She does not believe that cutting sugar out is necessary, but she is not particularly focused on hypoglycemia, either.

Atkins Diet

The Atkins Diet is followed by many hypoglycemics with success because the primary tenet of this diet is limiting the amount of carbohydrates we eat. As we saw in the discussion of the glycemic index, carbohydrates have the biggest effect on blood sugar.

The Atkins diet is primarily a weight loss diet. I believe that worrying about weight loss should be secondary to feeling healthy, but it is true that hypoglycemics tend to lose weight as their blood sugar stabilizes. Insulin is a storage hormone, and most hypoglycemics tend to have too much insulin floating around their systems. As the blood sugar stabilizes, the insulin production goes down, and most people will lose weight.

What I have seen is that many hypoglycemics do follow low carbohydrate diets. The amount of carbohydrate that can be tolerated seems to vary greatly from person to person, so this is very much a trial-and-error process for individual hypoglycemics.

Dr. Atkins was very critical of the mainstream preoccupation with high-carbohydrate, low-fat diets. Many studies do confirm that the high-carbohydrate, low-fat diets aren't working and it's clear that North Americans are fatter than ever before.

Although the Atkins diet works for many people, including many hypoglycemics, it doesn't ban sugar. For non-hypoglycemics who just want to lose weight, this is probably fine and won't cause any problems. Once you already have hypoglycemia, though, you probably need a stricter approach. But it should be said that if you follow Atkins to the letter, you probably won't be able to fit any sugar into your diet, at least in the "Induction Phase" of the plan.

Dr. Atkins' purpose was to "heal" the body's metabolism by changing it from glucose-burning to fat-burning. How quickly this metabolic change-over occurs will depend upon how strictly you follow the diet and how poorly your metabolism is working by the time you start to change how you eat.

Proponents of other diets, also concerned with healing the metabolism, still express concern that the Atkins diet restricts carbohydrates too much. The jury is still out on this, so the best thing to do is check with your own health care provider.

Exercising is an important part of the Atkins diet, and according to the book, you're not "doing Atkins" unless you exercise, too.

Zone Diet

The Zone diet is similar to the Atkins diet in that it is designed to control insulin levels by reducing carbohydrates. Operating without hunger and with a clear mind constitutes being in "the Zone", a state in which insulin is at the optimum level. Unlike Atkins, the Zone is not sold as a weight loss diet, although many of its adherents do report weight loss. The Zone diet does not subscribe to the extremely low carbohydrate approach of Atkins, and uses a diet plan consisting of "blocks" of protein, carbohydrate and fat in the recommended proportions. The Zone prescribes three meals and two snacks.

The Zone diet is used by lots of hypoglycemics—it seems to work well for many.

Krimmel Diet

The Krimmel diet plan is the only diet (that I know of) specifically developed for hypoglycemics. It follows the standard high carbohydrate, low fat paradigm with the significant difference that sugar is removed.

Like all other hypoglycemic diets, the ˙Krimmels recommend replacing all refined grains with whole grains.

The Schwarzbein Principle II

Dr. Diana Schwarzbein is an endocrinologist who has developed eating and lifestyle guidelines that, she claims, will re-balance the body's hormones and reverse ageing. Unlike the Atkins and Zone diets, she does not limit her attention to the action of insulin, but tracks adrenalin and cortisol as well. This is very appropriate for hypoglycemics (and probably many other people as well) since hypoglycemics often have "burned-out" adrenal glands. She does not focus on hypoglycemia in particular but like Dr. Atkins, her goal is to heal the metabolism.

Although the focus is not specifically centered on hypoglycemia, insulin resistance is addressed. The primary problems to solve in achieving balanced hormones, according to Dr. Schwarzbein, are insulin resistance and burned-out adrenal glands. Hypoglycemia is a metabolic illness and both of these problems are very common in hypoglycemics, so I believe that this diet could be very effective for hypoglycemics.

Weight loss is covered and discussed, but as a secondary goal. Once your metabolism is healed, Dr. Schwarzbein contends, you will naturally shed excess fat weight. She is very clear, though, in asserting that excess weight is a problem that is secondary to healing your metabolism. As she puts it, "Don't lose weight to be healthy, get healthy to lose weight".

Dr. Schwarzbein's approach is much more comprehensive than any of the others in that stress, exercise and sleep are also important components of the healing plan. While most of the plans advocate adding exercise to your lifestyle, Dr. Schwarzbein has seen many patients who exercise too much, a practice she considers as damaging as no exercise.

The diet itself is not a low-carbohydrate or a high-carbohydrate diet. It is moderate in all things, and advocates a balance of carbohydrates, proteins and healthy fats. It also advocates removing refined sugars and artificial sweeteners, alcohol, nicotine and caffeine ("toxic chemicals", she calls them). As I mentioned in an earlier chapter, all of these affect blood sugar levels, and should be avoided if you have hypoglycemia. Well, according to Dr. Schwarzbein, complete healing of your metabolism can't take place while you are still using any of these "toxic chemicals".

The South Beach Diet

The very popular South Beach Diet was developed by Dr. Arthur Agatston, M.D. to improve the health of his cardiac patients. He found that many of them were overweight and suffering from metabolic syndrome (prediabetes).

Dr. Agatston found that the standard high-carb, low fat diet just didn't have a long term positive effect on his patients' weight, cholesterol or tryglycerides. He really wanted to see an improvement in their blood chemistry.

The first two weeks of The South Beach Diet involves cutting out all bread, pasta, rice and fruit. Even sweet vegetables like carrots are off the list at first. And of course, all sugar has to go. The goal of the first two weeks is to reduce or eliminate your cravings for carbohydrates.

The main difference between The South Beach Diet and the Atkins diet is that for The South Beach Diet, saturated fats are limited. This means that proteins like bacon are limited, too.

As the diet continues, you can add back high fiber carbohydrates slowly and of course, you will never go back to your original level of consumption. The South Beach Diet is primarily concerned with weight loss and the improvement of blood chemistry with the goal of preventing heart disease.

The Ron Rosedale Diet

According to Dr. Ron Rosedale, hypoglycemia is just one step on the journey to poor health that includes insulin resistance and diabetes. He believes that our carbohydrate-rich diet is the primary cause of diabetes, heart disease and some cancers.

Dr. Rosedale has had great success turning around high blood pressure, heart disease and even cancer since the early '90's by prescribing a high fiber diet. Since high fiber food causes a slower insulin response, Dr. Rosedale's diet allows only high fiber carbohydrates and a moderate amount of protein. He describes his philosophy as "high-fat, adequate-protein, low-carbohydrate".

Unlike Dr. Atkins, Dr. Rosedale does not prescribe a limit on the grams of carbohydrate allowed, but simply specifies that all carbohydrates eaten must be high fiber carbohydrates. He does specify a protein limit. In general, the Rosedale diet specifies a ratio of approximately 15% carbohydrate, 25% protein, and 60% fat, but the book includes formulae for calculating the protein required for each individual's body size and shape. Modifications are made for diabetics and those who exercise heavily.

He believes that, to some degree, all North Americans are diabetic and that the low blood sugar symptoms we experience are a response to the level that each of us finds too low. He believes that the body can be conditioned to accept a much lower blood sugar level as "normal". He says that the symptoms have less to do with the absolute blood sugar level and everything to do with the level each individual's body is accustomed to.

Dr. Rosedale believes that sugar in all forms should be avoided, as should every food that readily turns into sugar.

He encourages light to moderate exercise in the form of weight training as a way to "work off" the carbohydrates that we have eaten, but that excessive exercise, an hour of jogging a day, for example, is actually bad for you.

Rosedale's Rules (paraphrased from *The Rosedale Diet*)

▋ Feel good about yourself: Enjoy the knowledge that you are undertaking a diet that will make you feel and look better than you have in years. Smile and feel good about taking this positive step.

▋ Avoid sugar and starch: Avoid potatoes, bread, pasta, cereal, corn and all grains for the first three weeks. After the first three weeks you can add the occasional slice of high fiber, low carb bread as long as this does not increase your cravings for more.

▋ Don't be afraid of fat, but eat good fat — Eat fat if you are hungry: Examples are nuts, avocados, fatty fish and olives.

▋ Limit saturated fat for the first three weeks: No beef, pork, lamb and most dairy products. After the first three weeks, you can add lean beef, lamb and pork, but if you want to continue to lose weight, you should minimize these.

■ Eat the right amount of protein for you: This is a high fat diet, not a high protein diet. Eat the right amount of protein for your body type. *The Rosedale Diet* supplies formulae for calculating the correct amount of protein for you.

■ Eat when you are hungry: Don't walk around hungry. When you are hungry, eat good fats, protein (if you haven't already exceeded your protein limit) and fiber (like vegetables)

■ Drink lots of water: Stick to water, seltzer or flavored water (tea and herbal teas). No soda of any type, even diet soda, and no juice.

■ Don't eat a lot at one time: Several small meals and snacks throughout the day are better for your metabolism than three large meals.

■ Eat slowly: If you eat slowly, your brain will get the message that you are filling up and you will know when it's time to stop eating.

■ Don't eat for at least three hours before bedtime: Your last meal of the evening should be at least 12 hours from your first meal in the morning. This gives your body the time it needs to rest and heal and this lets your digestive system rest, too.

■ Exercise after the last meal of the day (if possible): 15-20 minutes of mild resistance exercise or take a short uphill walk.

■ Don't slip up—at least for the first three weeks: It takes about three weeks for your metabolism to retool so that you switch from being a "sugar burner" to a "fat burner".

So many options—what should I eat?

With so many diets to choose from, it's difficult to figure out what you should be eating. So here are some rules of thumb:

▮ Choose lots of vegetables, and eat them raw as much as possible. If you cook them, steam them, but leave them crisp.

▮ Choose whole grains, and unprocessed, natural foods as much as possible.

▮ Add protein and fat to all your meals and snacks to slow your glycemic response to the carbohydrates that you eat.

▮ Cut back your serving sizes of potatoes, rice, pasta and breads. In the portions most of us consume, they are all a glycemic problem.

▮ Don't eat refined sugary foods and cut out all soft drinks.

▮ Switch to decaffeinated coffee and tea, or eliminate coffee and tea.

▮ Don't drink alcohol.

▮ Stop smoking.

Step by step—Changing your diet

If you are just starting to consider changing your diet, please don't think you have to do it all at once. Take it slowly. Let your body and your mind adjust to this new way of eating. I suggest making each of these steps last anywhere from a week to a couple of months. Use the Hypoglycemia Workbook at the back of this book to help you change your diet, and make the changes work for you.

Eat small amounts frequently

When you first begin changing your diet, start by eating more often.

Perhaps you already eat three fairly balanced meals almost every day, but sometimes you skip breakfast. Make your goal for this week to always eat breakfast. Once you have mastered that, plan for a snack between breakfast and lunch and another between lunch and supper. If you often sleep poorly, you may also want to plan a snack between supper and bedtime. Many hypoglycemics don't realize that their restlessness and excessively "vivid" dreaming is a symptom of low blood sugar during the night.

Getting started is the hardest part. Once you start to think in terms of snacking, you naturally begin to plan what you will eat. If you have been keeping a food journal, you are already getting an idea which foods work for you and which don't. It gets easier over time, so stick with it.

Make snacking a habit by doing it every day. When you have to be out, take an extra few minutes to think about what you will take with you so that you can snack at the usual time. I can't say enough about the benefits of nuts as an easy, convenient snack, and they are very portable, too. Almonds are particularly nutritious. (Nuts have protein, fat and carbohydrate.)

Choose balanced snacks and meals

Forget about low fat foods. Shocking, I know, but fats that occur naturally in "real" foods can be good for you. Everyone, but especially hypoglycemics, should be eating in a balanced way by making sure that every meal and snack includes a proportion of protein, carbohydrate and fat. Note that the carbohydrates don't have to come from breads and cereals. Vegetables contain carbohydrates, too. Many of the diets you can read about give prescribed amounts of carbohydrate, protein and fat, and use percentages to describe how much to eat, but that entails counting them. I believe asking people to count "somethings" whether it is calories or carbohydrate and fat grams, is the quickest way to drive people away from the diet plan. The goal here is to eat well for health and well being, not to follow some rigid eating plan.

Seeds are a wonderful food to add here. They are high in protein, but they are also relatively high in fat so many people avoid them, but they contain so many useful nutrients, it would be a shame to eliminate them. Besides, they taste great in salads and breads and add a lovely crunch.

Another point about low fat "foods" is that if you check labels, you will notice that the lower the fat, the higher the sugar. Sugar or other sweeteners are added to compensate for the reduction in flavor that comes with the reduction in fat. So when you check labels, reduce or eliminate sugar first, and don't worry about fat. That doesn't mean that you should go overboard. Moderation is still the best policy.

Switch to high fiber carbohydrates

With the changes you have already made, you have probably cut down the amount of carbohydrates you eat. Increasing your protein and fat will make your meals more satisfying so you may already be reducing your pasta or bread bingeing.

Take the next step—make the carbohydrates you eat really count. Use vegetables and whole grains more. When you do eat pasta, make it whole wheat or brown rice pasta and reduce your portions. Always eat pasta with protein, meat sauce and cheese, for example, and don't overcook the pasta. Al dente pasta (cooked past the "crunchy" point, but before the "mushy" point) breaks down more slowly in your system, so it won't raise your blood sugar as much.

When you eat bread or a bagel, make it whole grain and use half the amount you would normally eat. Then add a lovely coating of cream cheese or almond butter, and enjoy. You don't need to feel deprived just because the portions are smaller.

Whatever else you do, eat your vegetables. The best way to eat them is raw, but when you need them cooked, steam them and leave them a bit crunchy. You get more vitamins that way, and more fiber, too. The more fiber the better, since fiber lowers the glycemic index of the food and slows absorption into your system.

If you eat fruit, eat it raw, and with the skin. Avoid fruit juices. Juicing removes all the fiber, and makes your blood sugar soar. As a matter of fact, avoid drinking your meals at all. Drinking lots of fluids is great, but that just means that you should be drinking water with and between all your meals and snacks.

Avoid sugar (in all its forms)

Sugar, by definition, has a high glycemic index, and goes straight into your bloodstream. Fiber, protein and fat can slow sugar's progress and the resultant sugar and insulin

Table 3: Read labels and beware of hidden sugars. These are just some of the dozens of names that really just mean "sugar".

Barley malt/malted barley	Invert sugar
Beet sugar	Lactose
Black strap molasses	Levulose
Brown rice sugar	Malt
Brown rice syrup	Maltodextrin
Brown sugar	Maltose
Cane juice	Maple sugar
Cane sugar	Maple syrup
Cane syrup	Microcrystalline cellulose
Cane syrup solids	Molasses
Caramel	Natural sweeteners
Caramel coloring	Polydextrose
Confectioners' sugar	Powdered sugar
Corn sweetener	Raisin juice or syrup
Corn syrup	Raw sugar
Corn syrup solids	Rice syrup
Crystalline fructose	Simple syrup
Date sugar	Sorghum
Dextrin	Sucanat
Dextrose	Sucrose (White table sugar;
Disaccharide	50% glucose 50% fructose.)
Fructo-oligosaccharides	Sugar cane syrup
Fructose	Syrup
Fruit juice concentrate	Turbinado sugar
Galactose	Unrefined sugar
Glucose	
Glycerin	
Granulated sugar	
Hexitol	
High-fructose corn syrup	
Honey	

Source: This partial list was used with permission. Connie Bennett, www.SugarShock.com, Founder/Moderator, Yahoo kicksugar support group.

spikes, but is much easier to keep your blood sugar stable if you decide to avoid sugar as much as possible.

See Table 3 for dozens of names that really just mean "sugar".

As you can see, there are dozens of ways that manufacturers try to sneak sugar into processed food. It is best to avoid them all as much as possible.

All of the Protein bars I've seen, and even those sold under the Zone and Atkins names include sugar. The top ingredient in some of the Zone bars is brown rice syrup, aka sugar! (To be fair, although sugars appear on the ingredients list of the Atkins bars, the amounts are miniscule.)

Stevia is another sweetener that you will occasionally see on labels. This is not a sugar and has no effect on blood sugar, so it is safe for hypoglycemics. I still recommend against it, though. Your goal should be to get to the point where you no longer crave sweet foods, and as long as you are using any sweetener at all, you won't change your taste buds. If your taste buds lose their taste for sugar, you will find it much easier to stay away from harmful sugars.

Avoid caffeine

Caffeine, like sugar, causes an insulin response. And like sugar, it can be hidden in many foods, but you will be able to avoid it if you are informed and alert.

Caffeine is also addictive, so it may be difficult to stop grabbing for that cup of coffee or can of cola. I found that I used caffeine to mask my low sugar symptoms. When I felt rotten, I knew that my trusty diet cola would make me feel better. Out in the car, I always had my diet cola. After exercise—need that cola.

In addition to all that caffeine, I was also getting aspartame—too much of it. Recent studies have shown that artificial sweeteners, rather than helping you lose weight, actually *increase* your food cravings. Newsflash—"Diet foods containing aspartame can actually make you fatter!"

In addition to coffee and colas, caffeine appears in many other items like:

▮ Black tea (orange pekoe, Earl Grey...)

▮ Green tea

▮ Some soft drinks (examples are Mountain Dew (in the U.S.) and Jolt Cola)

▮ Chocolate

When you are first making the change, avoid decaffeinated teas and coffees. There isn't yet a process that can remove every last vestige of caffeine during the decaffeination process, and some hypoglycemics are bothered by even the smallest amount of caffeine. Swap your coffee and tea for herbal teas (I know, it seems a pretty poor substitute at first), and exchange your soft drinks for water. Even soft drinks that don't have any caffeine still have sugar or aspartame, and aren't a good choice for hypoglycemics.

Once you have "kicked" the caffeine habit, you may want to try a cup of decaf tea or coffee and take note of how you feel. Perhaps it will bother you, perhaps it won't but either way, use decaffeinated products in moderation. Even something that is fine when you have it a couple of times a week may not be fine if you have it twice a day.

As for chocolate, cut it out completely for at least the first two months of your new diet. If, after that, you still crave it, go for dark chocolate and make sure that it's organic. Dark chocolate contains much less sugar than milk chocolate, and buying organic ensures that you won't be getting any pesticides.

Avoid alcohol

Alcohol is essentially sugar to your body and can be dangerous to hypoglycemics. Mixed drinks are especially bad because they combine carbohydrates and sugar. Many hypoglycemics can't tolerate alcohol at all, but it may be hard at first to stop using it. Even if you aren't an alcoholic, drinking that nightly glass of wine may be a hard thing to stop simply because it has become a habit (plus a sugar boost!).

Anything that has become a habit, whether it is a physical addiction or a social habit can be difficult to change. Taking note of how alcohol makes you feel, and how you feel later may help you break the habit. If you always feel unwell just after a drink, or even the morning after, that will be an incentive to stop. This is another place that your food journal will help.

Start by cutting out all mixed drinks. This will lower your carbohydrate intake, thereby reducing your insulin response. Then try to cut down the number of drinks you have each time you have alcohol. If you normally would have two glasses of wine with dinner, cut back to one. If you would normally have three glasses of beer at the bar with your friends (before taking the cab home, of course) cut back to two. Every little bit helps, and you will find that it becomes easier. You may find that you feel better the morning after, even if you didn't feel you were drinking to excess before.

Quit smoking

If you need any more reasons to quit smoking, here is one more. Nicotine, like caffeine, has an effect on your blood sugar and will mask low blood sugar symptoms. That means that you will never get really good blood sugar control until you quit smoking.

I have never smoked, but that doesn't mean that I am unaware of how difficult it can be to quit. A man very close to me tried to quit many times over the four or five decades he smoked, and finally was able to kick the habit five years ago. It just takes the right incentive for most people, and when you realize just how much better you will feel after your blood sugar is stable, I hope you will be able to make this commitment to your health and your future. And don't be afraid to ask for help. Your doctor will have many suggestions for help in quitting smoking, and will be thrilled that you are up for the challenge.

Your diet

Pick and choose from the diets I've described and try the Hypoglycemia Workbook at the back of this book. If you find counting carbohydrates is easy and works, do that. If you would prefer to track the glycemic indices of the food you choose, that's good, too. Keep in mind that your needs will change over time, so revisit these steps every few months. A change that may seem impossible when you are starting out may seem do-able a few months in. It will feel great to realize that you are in control of your own health and well-being.

Make these changes as easy as possible on yourself, and remember: *Be patient with yourself.* You don't need any additional stresses to make life more challenging than it already is.

Diet Resources

Check out these references. We need to take help wherever we can get it!

Agatston, Arthur. *The South Beach Diet.* New York: Rodale, 2003

Brand-Miller, Jennie, Ph.D., T.M.S. Wolever, M.D., Ph.D., S. Colagiuri, M.D., K. Foster-Powell, M.Nutr. & Diet. *The Glucose Revolution.* New York: Marlowe & Company, 1999

Atkins, Robert. C., M.D. *Dr. Atkins New Diet Revolution.* New York. M. Evans and Company, 2002

Schwarzbein, Diana, M.D. *The Schwarzbein Principle II.* Deerfield Beach, Florida: Health Communications Inc., 2002

Krimmel, Patricia, E.A. Krimmel, P.T. Krimmel. *The Low Blood Sugar Cookbook.* Bryn Mawr, PA: Franklin Publishers, 1986

Sears, Barry, MD. *The Zone.* New York: Harper Collins Regan Books, 2000

Rosedale, Ron and Carol Coleman. *The Rosedale Diet.* New York: HarperCollins Publishers, Inc., 2004

Chapter 8

Will I still live to be 120?

■ ■ ■ ■ Pete's Story

I think I have had hypoglycemia all my life. I remember passing out in the sixth grade, and I'm sure that it was due to low blood sugar. I have always suffered from ADD (Attention Deficit Disorder), so school was never easy for me. I've also had trouble with depression on and off for most of my life.

As a teen in the late 1950's, I spent some time in the Coast Guard in Cape May, New Jersey. I didn't do well there, and I would pass out in the early morning. I think it had a lot to do with the Kool-Aid we were given three times a day. I was treated for epilepsy and discharged.

I first heard about hypoglycemia from my mother, who was also hypoglycemic. She and I read the first work written about hypoglycemia by Dr. Seale. My son is also hypoglycemic and has the same learning problems and ADD that I have always struggled with.

My father came from a family of sugar importers; a bit ironic, actually. I think my dad was probably hypoglycemic, too, since he always had trouble with alcohol. He was a newspaperman, not an easy profession if you need regular meals, and the newspaper business certainly seemed to involve a lot of alcohol in those days.

I was diagnosed with hypoglycemia after a six-hour GTT (glucose tolerance test) in about 1968. At one point, my blood sugar went down to 55. The doctor told me to eat more protein but that was all I learned from him. He said nothing about nutrition. Then, about 15 or 20 years ago, an endocrinologist told me to follow the diabetic diet. At the time, that consisted of no sugar, moderate amounts of protein and lots of carbohydrate.

I worked for many years as a window clerk for the Post Office. It was an incredibly stressful position and I eventually had to give it up for a less stressful responsibility. The people at the post office really didn't understand the problems I was having, and I eventually had to opt for early retirement.

In the past few years, I've had to deal with low thyroid, rheumatoid arthritis and prostate problems, and I decided to have all my amalgam fillings removed about nine years ago. I am currently undergoing chelation therapy for mercury poisoning. Each expensive treatment involves three hours of being hooked up to an IV. I have also been diagnosed with the Epstein Barr virus.

Over the years, I found another specialist for help with my hypoglycemia, and she did regular GTT's, after the first one, to track the success of treatments. Glucose tolerance tests are very difficult to get through and I found this very stressful.

I manage my hypoglycemia fairly well now. My whole family gets up for breakfast at 4:00 am. My wife and son go back to bed for a few hours, though. I make my own yogurt and I am experimenting with making kefir. Both are great for replacing intestinal flora, and a healthy digestive system really helps with the hypoglycemia. I also take chromium and acidophilus. I stay away from sugar and all other sweeteners, although I did a little experimenting with Stevia. I also avoid all soy products.

I'm retired now, and I spend a lot of time on the Internet researching hypoglycemia and my related problems and I do a lot of reading. I receive newsletters from the Westin A. Price Foundation website and the Dr. Williams newsletter. One of my favorite new books is the latest revision of the Saunders/Ross book.

Pete is retired and lives in Little Silver, New Jersey

What about the future?

So you have hypoglycemia or you strongly suspect you do. What does this mean for the future? That depends on what **you** do about it. If you do nothing, you are inviting diabetes and heart disease.

As we discussed in an earlier chapter, hypoglycemics are often insulin resistant. Insulin resistance tends to increase as you get older and leads to high cholesterol and high triglycerides—the infamous Syndrome X.

Hypoglycemia is an indication that your metabolism is not working as well as it should be. Your metabolism is affected by many things—everything from genetics to exercise, stress and diet. When you were twenty, you could probably eat almost anything, drink quite a lot, deprive yourself of sleep and manage large stresses. This could have led you to believe that you're not affected by your diet or lifestyle. But now you have hypoglycemia and you've probably also put on some weight. Even though you are eating better and maybe sleeping more than you did in college, you've started having all these disturbing symptoms.

As we age, our bodies become less able to cope with the stresses we place on them. First of all, as we age, our metabolic systems are less resilient, and it's more difficult to mask the effects of poor habits. Second, the damage we are doing now is adding to the damage we did in college, or perhaps even before that. The bad habits are adding up and actually making us age faster than we should. This puts us on the path to diabetes and heart disease.

This is your wake-up call. You can continue as you are, dizzy, unable to concentrate, eating constantly, or you can decide to make a change. Start with the diet suggestions found in this book, and make small improvements. Eating sugar-free will not always be a smooth path, and it will take time to see the full effects, but it will improve your health and probably increase your lifespan.

Does this mean I will become diabetic?

Having hypoglycemia doesn't have to lead to diabetes.

Keep in mind that we are only talking about Type II diabetes. Ninety-five percent of diabetes sufferers have Type II diabetes. The other five percent that have Type I diabetes have suffered a complete, spontaneous failure of the pancreas, often in their childhood. Type I diabetics inject insulin to maintain a constant blood sugar level. Type II diabetics can often use oral medication in addition to their dietary modifications.

Hypoglycemia occurs when your body is producing too much insulin. In addition to all of the other problems that too much insulin can cause (overweight and heart disease), producing extra insulin all the time causes great wear and tear on your pancreas. Type II diabetes results when your pancreas can no longer keep up with your body's insulin demands.

When this happens, it produces less insulin, or sometimes the insulin produced isn't as effective as it once was. Type II diabetes used to be a disease of middle-age, but it is now occurring more often in people much younger, some even as young as their teens. Having diabetes can mean increased risk of heart disease, stroke, blindness and foot gangrene leading to amputation.

Not all hypoglycemics end up diabetic, but you have a good chance if you don't change your lifestyle, especially if there is diabetes in your family. Even if you feel that the diet is too strict or your symptoms aren't that bad, is it really worth the risk?

Will the hypoglycemia get worse as I get older?

The longer you abuse your body with poor diet, too little sleep and too much stress, the more the damage builds up. In addition, as your body ages, your system no longer absorbs nutrients from your food as well as it did before.

With these two factors in play, yes, your hypoglycemia will get worse as you age, but **only if** you do nothing about it.

You have a choice. If you choose to do nothing, your symptoms are likely to get worse and you are more likely to fall into the chronic diseases of ageing so common in this century. But diabetes and heart disease are not inevitable.

It is never too late to make a change that will improve your life and your enjoyment of it. When you choose to change your diet and lifestyle, you will see an improvement in how you feel and over time, I predict that you will also feel younger. Both Drs. Rosedale and Schwarzbein believe that you can reduce your body's internal age over time by changing your diet and lifestyle.

Here is a sample success story from the files of Dr. Ron Rosedale at the International Center for Metabolic and Longevity Medicine:

> *This patient [...] saw me one afternoon and said that he had literally just signed himself out of the hospital "AMA," or "Against Medical Advice". Like in the movies, he had ripped out his IV's. The next day he was scheduled to have his second by-pass surgery. He had been told that if he did not follow through with this by-pass surgery, within two weeks he would be dead. He couldn't walk from the car to the office without severe chest pain. He was on 102 units of insulin and his blood sugars were 300 plus. He was on eight different medications for various things. But his first by-pass surgery was such a miserable experience he said he would rather just die than have to go through the second one and had heard that I might be able to prevent that. To make a long story short, this gentleman right now is on no insulin. I first saw him three and a half years ago. He plays golf four or five times a week. He is on no medications whatsoever, he has no chest pain, and he has not had any surgery. He started an organization called "Heart Support of America" to educate people that there are alternatives to by-pass surgery that have nothing to do with surgery or medication. That organization, he last told me had a mailing list of over a million people.*

If Dr. Rosedale can effect a dramatic turnaround like this by changing a heart patient's diet, imagine what it can do for you.

I'm overweight—Is this a cause or an effect?

Hypoglycemics often have chronically high levels of insulin in their systems. Insulin is a storage hormone and instructs your body what to do with the food you take in. If there is too much sugar for immediate use, you will store some in your liver, but most of it will be stored as fat.

Over time, this can really build up and you can find yourself much heavier than your ideal weight.

I would suggest that forcing yourself to endure yet another diet is not the way to go. Concentrate your energy on healing your metabolism and stop worrying about fat and calories, at least for a while. Work on improving your diet, removing sugar and refined foods. Plan ways to reduce your stress and get more sleep. As your metabolism heals, chances are good that your body will begin to move naturally to its ideal weight.

In *The Schwarzbein Principle II*, Dr. Schwarzbein warns that, depending on the starting state of your metabolism, you might actually *gain* weight before beginning to lose it. Don't panic—stick with the hypoglycemic diet!

There is an ideal hormone balance that your body is always trying to achieve. As long as you are abusing your body with too much sugar and too little fiber, too much stress and too little sleep, your body just can't do it. Only when you change your habits and start to heal can your body begin to catch up and sometimes that entails putting on some weight. As the healing continues, your body will also tend toward your ideal composition and the weight will go. Whatever happens, don't be tempted to crash diet. Stick to your healthy eating. It **will** pay off.

It's important to mention here that a significant number of hypoglycemics are underweight, and have difficulty keeping weight on. The solution is the same. Level your blood sugar and your weight should begin to normalize.

I know I sound like a heretic, but make your weight a secondary concern. Start by healing your metabolism by controlling your blood sugar. I promise that it will be worth the effort.

How long should I keep up the new diet?

After the sugar tirade in Chapter 4, it may seem clear to you that the removal of sugar and refined foods from your diet should be a more-or-less permanent lifestyle change. And the diet chapter talked a lot about changes to your lifestyle as well. Cut out smoking, drinking, get enough sleep, and eat at least six times a day. But how long until you are cured?

It may take you a month; it make take you two years, but you will probably feel "cured" at some point. You may find that you never have symptoms any more, even when you eat more carbohydrates than usual or even when you eat a dessert now and then. You may notice that you don't have to eat as often, and that you feel strong and energetic almost all the time.

Does this mean that you can go back to eating as you did?

Remember how you got into trouble with hypoglycemia in the first place. Having a stronger, healthier system allows you to eat a quality diet with a few cheats. Going back to the diet that caused the problem in the first place will reverse all of the progress you have made.

Your metabolic problems were caused by poor diet and lifestyle, and even after you feel "cured", you won't be able to go back to the same abuse. If you go back to your old diet and lifestyle, it may take a couple of months or even a bit longer, but your hypoglycemia will come back, along with all of the risks that you changed your diet to avoid.

The good news (in addition to you feeling great) is that your tastes will change. After some months on your new diet, you will find that very sweet foods no longer taste good. This is why you should avoid artificial sweeteners—it is better to train your taste buds away from sweet tastes. One of the problems you probably had when your hypoglycemia was at its worst was food cravings. Once you have your blood sugar under control your cravings will be rare, so you won't even be tempted to eat the foods you used to. And you won't be hungry all the time, so it will be much easier to avoid over-eating.

This doesn't mean that you will ever be able to ignore your diet. What it does mean is that your new eating style will become habit, and you'll be able to stop thinking about it all the time.

Will I have a normal lifespan?

Normal—what's that? I don't know, but I do know that if you get your blood sugar under control and you work on healing your metabolism, you are much less likely to die of one of the chronic diseases of ageing.

Some experts theorize that that the human body is capable of living to about 120 years before wearing out. Who knows? If we didn't have hardening of the arteries, diabetes, high blood pressure and heart disease, maybe we would live to be closer to 120. Think about all the things you could do with 100 healthy years!

If you could prevent or reduce all of these conditions by turning around your hypoglycemia now, wouldn't you do it?

Long term damage or long life: It's your choice.

Change is hard—procrastination is easy. So go back to the diet chapter and decide to take one baby step today. I promise it will be worth it.

Chapter 9

Other conditions that may affect me

■■■■*Sigrid's Story*

I have alimentary hypoglycemia. My symptoms started right after my stomach surgery, but the story doesn't start there.

In my teens, I was hyperthyroid, but even with medication, I wasn't keeping it under control, so at age 17, I had a subtotal thyroidectomy. I could eat and drink anything, and I smoked and drank a lot of coffee. Then, in 1981, a bad car accident left me with 13 broken bones and a collapsed lung—the steering wheel had gone right into my abdomen. These problems continued as I developed a hiatus hernia and fourth degree ulcers. The first stomach surgery was botched and so it failed to correct the problem—I was still vomiting every day. I decided to see another surgeon, and he warned me that he might have to cut my vagus nerve (vagotomy) in order to be able to correct the problem. I was absolutely against this, but he refused to do the initial surgery unless I signed the release. When I awoke in the recovery room, the vagotomy had been done.

That's when the real trouble began. I had wild mood swings, from tears to happiness to rage. I was diagnosed with hypothyroidism— a complete reversal of my previous condition—and I was exhausted all the time.

161

I went from doctor to doctor, including psychological professionals for eight years, getting diagnosed with everything from fibromyalgia to stress and depression. Anti-depressants just made me feel worse. By 1996, I was passing out, falling over and walking into things. I often hyperventilated and my speech was slurred. I was spending all of my time on the couch.

More testing revealed that I had a B12 deficiency, which explained my sleepiness and exhaustion, but the endocrinologist also sent me for a five-hour glucose tolerance test. The result of the first blood test, non-fasting, was 2.5 (normal is 5-6). After the first hour of the test, my insulin level was 3397—22 times more than the normal level! At the 2-hour mark, my blood sugar measured 1.6. It was so low that I fell asleep and I was given juice to allow me to finish the test. Looking back, I should have refused to finish the test, but I was feeling so low that I couldn't even think straight, much less make a decision.

After the test, I felt sick for five days, but I did end up with a diagnosis of hypoglycemia.

In the years since then, I have tried many diets, including the Krimmel diet, [Dr.] Harvey Ross's diet, and a modified Atkins diet.

Although the Atkins diet worked better than the others, I still had no energy, so I now eat 60-80g of carbohydrate each day. I have always had food allergies, but since getting hypoglycemia, I have also become allergic to pollens, grasses, dust, feathers and many foods, including dairy, nuts and soy. The only protein left to me is meat. I've tried many vegetables, but I have also developed acute reactions to pesticides and cannot eat any vegetables at all except for well-cooked cauliflower and broccoli.

I take antihistamines and get allergy shots, but they cause me problems every day because of the alcohol and sugars they contain.

Hypoglycemia is made much more difficult to manage with all of these allergies, and it has created a terrible void and a feeling of loss for me because food satisfies emotional and social needs and is often celebratory.

My diet is very limited—I eat only about 12 different foods, and I still can't get away from all of the foods that cause allergic reactions. I have symptoms whether I eat large or small meals.

I was eating a lot of sugar-free bacon because it was an additional protein that I could eat and it helped me keep some weight on. I'm 5'9" and I usually weighed only 120 pounds. When I ate bacon every day, I was able to maintain a weight of 132 pounds. With the additional carbohydrate I am now eating to improve my energy, I have gained weight and I am now struggling with being heavier than I want to be.

I still eat eggs for breakfast and 2 servings of nuts per day. I get sick of meat and poultry, but I have also cut out fish because I have suffered from mercury poisoning. I break my diet only every 3-4 months, but I always pay for it by feeling bad for a few days afterward. I find myself thinking about food all the time and I am always hungry.

In spite of all my efforts, I'm not well but I have not lost hope. I will continue to work at finding a diet and medications that will give me my life back. I know that I have to be able to feel better than I do. I just won't give up.

Sigrid is an author and freelance editor living in Ottawa, Canada.

There's more?

You would think that dealing with hypoglycemia is enough for any one person, but for many people, hypoglycemia is only part of the picture. Hypoglycemia often shows up with other conditions and it really muddies the waters when it comes to diagnosis. Most hypoglycemics aren't as severely challenged as Sigrid is, but many of us do have a combination of conditions. Some are linked, but cause and effect are almost impossible to figure out. In some cases, the conditions that have set us up for hypoglycemia have also weakened our immune system, making us more susceptible to other problems, allergies, for instance.

This chapter will list many of the conditions often seen in conjunction with hypoglycemia and provide information, where it exists, about how they are linked.

Dr. Diana Schwarzbein, in her book *The Schwarzbein Principle II*, says that hypoglycemia (among other things) can cause a reduction in the production of serotonin, and it is the low level of serotonin that contributes to a nasty list of problems including:

▌ Attention Deficit Disorder (ADD) and Attention Deficit Hyperactivity Disorder (ADHD)
▌ Depression
▌ Chronic Fatigue Syndrome
▌ Fibromyalgia
▌ Irritable Bowel Syndrome
▌ Migraine headaches

▌ Menstruation problems and Premenstrual Syndrome (PMS)

▌ Seasonal Affective Disorder

The following paragraphs describe and discuss each of the above conditions. Each section outlines the symptoms and causes (if they are known). Although not all show explicit links to hypoglycemia, it is clear that hypoglycemia often accompanies them (or vice versa).

Attention Deficit Disorder (ADD) and Attention Deficit Hyperactivity Disorder (ADHD)

Most of us have heard of ADD and ADHD, and know children and adults affected. People with these disorders have trouble controlling their impulses and have to work very hard to "filter out" distractions. It often manifests itself in a school setting when a child seems unable to sit still and concentrate.

Although not all sources agree on the link between ADD, ADHD and hypoglycemia, most agree that diet can play a huge role in controlling symptoms and behavior. In addition to the sugar and caffeine links to ADD and ADHD, it has been found that many affected children react to combinations of food additives and chemicals.

Depression

There is a great deal of anecdotal evidence that hypoglycemia and depression are linked, and many hypoglycemics are taking anti-depressants or have taken them in the past.

165

This could be because many doctors misdiagnose hypoglycemia as mental illness, or because there really is a cause-effect relationship between the two. I believe that the true answer is a combination of these, and that where hypoglycemia exists, diet—not anti-depressants—is the best place to begin. There will, of course, be instances where anti-depressants will be necessary as well.

It has been documented that "Patients with hypoglycemia (low blood sugar) exhibit higher depression scores in response to glucose administration than those with normal blood sugar levels". This testing was done with diabetic patients with short-term episodes of hypoglycemia, but it appears that low blood sugar results in the patient being more likely to feel "low". Another source states that hypoglycemia causes depression, including the depression occurring with PMS.

If short-term episodes of low blood sugar can cause feelings of depression, chronic low blood sugar can probably cause long-term depression. Some practitioners still don't believe that depression EVER has a biological cause. Even if this is true, which seems doubtful, depression caused by discouragement about not feeling physically well, common in hypoglycemics, will still be improved by a reduction in hypoglycemia symptoms.

Chronic Fatigue Syndrome

Difficult as it is to diagnose, chronic fatigue syndrome (CFS) is considered as a diagnosis if the fatigue is severe enough to restrict daily activity by at least 50 percent, as long as all psychiatric causes have been eliminated.

A list of possible causes includes the Epstein-Barr virus (EBV), anemia, arthritis, chronic mercury poisoning from amalgam dental fillings, hypothyroidism, infection with the fungus candida albicans, sleep problems and hypoglycemia. It is fairly common for sufferers of CFS to also have intestinal parasites.

Nutritional deficiencies, allergies, thyroid dysfunction, candida, anemia and stress all can contribute to CFS.

Fibromyalgia

Fibromyalgia is condition of fatigue accompanied by unexplained muscle aches and pains. There is no definitive test for fibromyalgia, and it is often misdiagnosed at first. Distinctive to fibromyalgia is the presence of certain "tender points", eighteen points on the body that are particularly sensitive to the touch. Most people diagnosed with fibromyalgia are female and a significant number are disabled by the condition. Fibromyalgia and chronic fatigue syndrome are very similar with the main difference being that, in fibromyalgia, the muscle pain predominates over fatigue. In chronic fatigue syndrome, fatigue is the dominant complaint.

In both, the immune system is compromised and sufferers are prone to pick up opportunistic infections. Also in both, allergies and environmental sensitivities are common.

The course of fibromyalgia is unpredictable. Some people improve, others have periodic remissions of the condition and for many others the condition becomes chronic. The causes are also not known, although fibromyalgia has been linked to a history of clinical depression.

Other possible causes proposed in the literature include infection with the Epstein-Barr virus (EBV), the virus that causes infectious mononucleosis, candida albicans, chronic mercury poisoning from amalgam dental fillings, anemia, parasites, hypothyroidism and hypoglycemia.

Irritable Bowel Syndrome

Irritable bowel syndrome, or IBS, is a condition of the gastrointestinal tract. It is not a disease, but a set of symptoms, existing together, that cannot be explained by structural or chemical problems. Other names for IBS include "spastic colon", "spastic colitis", "mucus colitis" and "nervous stomach".

My search yielded very little information about a link between hypoglycemia and IBS, but interestingly, the treatments are similar. In both cases a high fiber diet, no caffeine, small frequent meals and reduced stress are recommended.

Migraine headaches

Headaches are a very common symptom of hypoglycemia, and in a 1957 study published in Brazil by Dr. Stephen Gyland, it was found that over 70 percent of hypoglycemics have headaches and migraines.

It is interesting to note that the National Headache Foundation has a hypoglycemia page, and it talks about migraines and accompanying carbohydrate cravings in some patients. Other sources list headaches and migraines resulting from causes as varied as food allergies and gastrointestinal problems such as too much yeast or too little stomach acid.

Menstruation disorders and PMS

Many sources note a link, depressed serotonin levels, between PMS and hypoglycemia, but only Dr. Schwarzbein ventures an explanation. Many of the sites do suggest that a change to a less-refined diet and increased exercise will be helpful in lessening the symptoms.

Many also suggest that taking anti-depressants will reduce the symptoms. Given that depression is another serotonin-linked problem, it isn't surprising that PMS and depression could occur together in some women.

Seasonal affective disorder (SAD)

Seasonal affective disorder, most commonly known as SAD, is a condition of depression during the dark months. Most sufferers feel low or depressed during the winter months when it is colder, there are fewer hours of sunlight, and they spend less time outside.

There is almost nothing in the literature to link SAD to hypoglycemia, other than Dr. Schwarzbein's reference, although one source suggests that hypoglycemia be ruled out before making a diagnosis of SAD. SAD often responds well to light therapy, and there is little documentation to suggest that SAD would respond to a change in diet.

Other conditions that have been linked to hypoglycemia include:

■ Candida albicans overgrowth

■ Hypothyroidism

■ Alcoholism

■ Nicotine addiction

■ Food allergies

■ Polycystic ovarian syndrome (PCOS)

■ Menier's syndrome

■ Obesity

■ Degenerative changes in kidneys

■ Stress

Candida albicans overgrowth

Candida is the most common yeast that occurs naturally in our gastrointestinal system. It is supposed to be there and we wouldn't do well without it. The problem occurs when the bacteria that normally keep it in check are compromised, and we end up with too much candida.

This can be, and often is, caused by taking antibiotics. Many of the meats we eat can contain antibiotics, too. Broad spectrum antibiotics that we might take for an ear infection, for instance, kill off not only the bacteria that caused the ear infection, but also many of the bacteria that keep our intestinal yeast under control. Ever notice that a vaginal yeast infection or oral thrush often follows a course of antibiotics? This is a signal that too many of the "good" bacteria were killed off along with the "bad".

Most of the time, our systems will recover and return to some kind of balance. For some people, however, this doesn't happen, and the candida takes over.

When this happens, you will notice frequent fungus infections like thrush and athletes foot, and you may have an increase in skin rashes as well. You may have recurrent vaginitis, bladder infections or prostatitis, and you may become sensitive to tobacco, perfume, chemical odors or auto exhaust fumes. Some people even report confusion, fatigue, poor memory, and depression.

Because yeast feeds on sugar (that's why yeast breads need sugar to rise), you may experience cravings for sweets, breads or alcoholic beverages.

It's not clear that candida overgrowth causes hypoglycemia, but if you give in to the sweets cravings that go along with it, your hypoglycemia symptoms will be aggravated.

Hypothyroidism

A friend told me one day that she had just been diagnosed with a hypothyroid condition. Curious, I asked her what that meant. What are the symptoms? Her answer was short and to the point. "You get fat and stupid."

This is extreme, but it's not surprising that she would feel that way. Reduced function of the thyroid does often result in weight gain and poorer concentration.

The thyroid is a small gland located in the neck. When the thyroid gland isn't working properly, you have a decreased metabolic rate, reduced food assimilation and depressed activity of other glands in the body.

Some of the symptoms are weight gain, chronic fatigue, fibromyalgia, frequent illness, feeling cold all the time, heart and arterial disease and depression or "the blues".

Hypoglycemia is linked to your insulin production. You will likely have hypoglycemia symptoms if you are producing too much insulin. Insulin also controls a lot of what goes on in the liver, and the liver also performs functions on the thyroid products (most notably T3 and T4), so if there are insulin problems, there are also likely to be problems with processing of the thyroid hormones.

When the insulin levels are brought back to normal, the thyroid levels can also return to the normal range.

Alcoholism

Excessive alcohol intake can cause incidents of hypoglycemia, and these are among the most dangerous, sometimes resulting in coma and even death.

There are medical professionals who have come to believe that hypoglycemia can also be a cause of alcoholism. Some studies have indicated that over 90 percent of alcoholics are hypoglycemics. While some of us crave candy or sweet carbohydrates, others use alcohol. Because many alcoholics forego eating in preference to alcohol, there are often deficiencies in many vitamins that would otherwise lessen the impact of low blood sugar.

There are reports of alcoholics who were able to get sober and stay sober for prolonged periods by adopting the hypoglycemia diet. This was found to be much more effective if the hypoglycemia sufferer was also able to give up caffeine and cigarettes.

Nicotine addiction

Like caffeine, nicotine causes an adrenaline reaction that pulls glucose from storage to meet the immediate (emergency) needs. It's easy to understand how difficult it could be for a hypoglycemia sufferer to stop smoking.

Nicotine often masks the symptoms of hypoglycemia, since the low blood sugar symptoms trigger the "need" for a cigarette. Nicotine withdrawal causes hypoglycemia symptoms, and weight gain can follow if sugary foods replace cigarettes when the low blood sugar cravings hit.

Food allergies

Many hypoglycemics also have food allergies and many people with food allergies have hypoglycemia. It's just not clear whether one causes the other. Some sources say that allergic reactions can cause hypoglycemia, but there are no studies to prove it.

What does seem clear is that many hypoglycemics also suffer from food allergies, perhaps because both can be symptoms of a compromised immune system.

It has also been suggested that hypoglycemia indicates a sensitivity or allergy to sugar. Depending on your definition of allergy, perhaps you could look at it this way. After all, if being sensitive to a food means that you have symptoms of some kind after eating it, perhaps hypoglycemics can be said to be "allergic" to sugar and refined carbohydrates.

Food allergies are strange. In many cases, craving for a particular food can indicate sensitivity to that food. When I heard that, my first thought was "Does this mean that I'm allergic to chocolate? Oh, Nooooo!" I also used to be a bread and cookie addict and I have discovered that I do have a wheat sensitivity. I have often thought that I was acting like a "sugar addict".

The most common food allergies are to dairy, wheat, eggs, corn, peanuts, yeast and soy. It has been estimated that most of us suffer from food sensitivities and that they are the underlying cause for many conditions usually treated by psychiatric means; for example, hyperactivity, attention deficit disorder (ADD) and schizophrenia.

Orthomolecular psychiatry clinics are springing up in the US, and they are showing success in treating otherwise resistant psychiatric cases using a combination of elimination of allergens and mega-doses of vitamins. The Huxley Institute has found that 60 percent of their schizophrenic patients suffer from hypoglycemia, as do 80 percent of those suffering from manic depression.

Most allergic reactions are somewhat easier to manage, but can run the gamut from respiratory symptoms (hay fever, asthma, sore throat), digestive discomfort (gastroenteritis, irritable bowl syndrome, celiac disease, diarrhea, constipation), cerebral problems (headaches, dizziness, sleep disorders, irritability, depression), skin-related problems (dermatitis, eczema, hives, rashes), or even seemingly unrelated disorders like arthritis, overweight, underweight, PMS or fatigue.

Treatment programs for the elimination of allergies abound on the Internet. Most are vitamin and mineral programs ("Buy our vitamins!") but I even saw one site offering laser therapy for the permanent elimination of allergic reactions.

The most usual treatment is to stop eating the offending food or by otherwise avoiding the allergen. In some food allergies, once the body has been cleared of the offending food, you may begin to be able to tolerate small amounts of the food once again. In other cases, even tiny amounts of the food might always cause a problem. Gluten allergies fall into this category. You will just have to stay away from the food permanently.

Caution: If you know you have an allergy to peanuts (for example) that causes an anaphylactic reaction, don't ever try to reintroduce peanuts to your diet. It's really not worth risking death to have one more taste!

Polycystic Ovarian Syndrome (PCOS)

Polycystic Ovarian Syndrome, or PCOS, is a condition in women with symptoms remarkably similar to those of hypoglycemia, with the added problems of ovarian cysts, infertility, male pattern hair growth and, strangely, male pattern baldness. Periods become irregular or disappear completely.

As with hypoglycemia, one of the primary tests done to diagnose PCOS is the glucose tolerance test because PCOS sufferers show elevated insulin levels. PCOS sufferers also often show elevated levels of testosterone and other male hormones, and that accounts for the male pattern hair growth and male pattern baldness.

It is believed that up to 30 percent of women suffer from PCOS to some degree. There is no cure, although many women must have the ovarian cysts surgically removed.

The most effective treatment of the other symptoms, though, is a change in diet. The International Council on Infertility Information Dissemination (INCIID) recommends reducing carbohydrate intake and increasing exercise. Although there is no cure for PCOS, the council notes that weight loss (most people suffering from PCOS are overweight) can really make a difference to the severity of the symptoms.

Menier's syndrome

Menier's syndrome or Menier's disease is a condition that causes vertigo, hearing loss, tinnitus (ringing in the ears) and a feeling of fullness in the affected ear(s). The severity of the symptoms can range from mild and infrequent to completely debilitating.

The causes are unknown, but everything from a knock on the head to food allergies to yeast overgrowth have been suggested.

The usual course of treatment is to limit salt in the diet. There are also lots of drugs used to treat Menier's but none of them works for everyone. The most extreme treatment is surgery to disconnect the balance mechanism, and this is only used in cases where the sufferer's dizziness and nausea are so severe that the person is unable to function. None of these treatments is a cure, however, and sufferers must learn to cope as they can, experimenting with various diets and other treatments.

There have been no definitive studies, but there have been reports that hypoglycemia is more common in people with Menier's than in the general population, and that the syndrome sometimes responds to a sugar-free, low-carbohydrate diet.

Obesity

Although there are many hypoglycemics who are underweight, the majority are overweight, some significantly. Along with high blood pressure, high cholesterol and diabetes, obesity is one of the group of conditions now called "Syndrome X". Syndrome X is the culmination of years of poor blood sugar control and poor diet.

Weight loss is crucial to the reversal of insulin resistance and Syndrome X. The good news is that getting your blood sugar under control often results in weight loss without additional effort.

Degenerative changes in kidneys

Chronic kidney disease is very common in diabetes. It is caused by blood vessel damage from the chronic high blood pressure that is often seen in diabetes. High blood pressure is also seen as hypoglycemia advances toward diabetes, so kidney damage is just one more avoidable (usually) side effect of uncontrolled blood sugar.

Stress

This is probably the least studied, but the most understood condition common to hypoglycemics. Stress has been found by many hypoglycemics to make their symptoms worse, probably because stress activates the adrenal gland, and chronic stress can cause adrenal burnout.

Adrenal problems often accompany hypoglycemia because incidents of low blood sugar activate the adrenals, and this overuse can lead to adrenal burnout.

On the other hand, stress and hypoglycemia symptoms are part of a vicious cycle. Stress can cause increased hypoglycemia symptoms and increased symptoms can lead to increased stress. Adrenal burnout is quite common in chronic hypoglycemics and adrenal gland healing is part of the hypoglycemia recovery process.

Combinations of conditions like the ones in this chapter really complicate diagnosis and treatment of all of them. Even when you have other conditions that cause or are caused by your hypoglycemia, you will still feel better when you change your diet, increase your exercise and sleep and reduce your stress. You can make a difference!

Chapter 10

How can I talk to my health care professionals?

■■■■Irene's story as told by her daughter

From my mother's diaries

1973 July: Glucose tolerance test

1973 September: Visit to Dr. J. Gay (inconclusive)

1973 October: Started hypoglycemic diet (ed.: I think this involved lots of small protein meals, no sweets, starches, alcohol, etc) diet continues through October (ed.: she finds it discouraging)

1973 December: To Dr. Gay—Verdict very good. Easy on carbohydrates.

1974: Saw Dr. J. Gilka, Ottawa (ed: female Ottawa doctor specializing in nutrition and holistic medicine)

1974 March: To see Dr. Paul Cutler—orthomolecular specialist, Ottawa

1974 September: Passed out during birthday dinner. Insulin shock.

1975 January: Went to lecture on hypoglycemia given by Dr. Gilka.

1975 March: Saw Dr. Gilka again.

I can remember Mummy always being tired and having a nap every afternoon while we were at school. She was very moody and irritable and went up and down a lot. She had always suffered from depression. She also got shaky when she needed sugar. I have to admit that we never made any connections, although she probably did. I think she finally found a holistic-type GP in Toronto who sent her for a glucose tolerance test and discovered that she was off the chart. Around the same time (or as a result?), she got into vitamins and health food in a big way, and started eating smaller, more frequent protein meals—and taking mega-vitamins. She often said that she would never have been able to go into real estate (which she did after my brother married) if she hadn't been on that treatment, because she just wouldn't have had the energy.

After she was diagnosed and changed her diet, her life changed and we all noticed it. She had far more energy, was able to actually get a job (in real estate) and do well at it, and seemed much less depressed and moody.

From my mother's "Chronology of Changes" written in 1988

1945: "Developed emotionally crippling trance-like state which persisted, in spite of every possible medical opinion, for twenty-eight years. (Eventually diagnosed, in Ottawa, as hypoglycemia and cured in three months by nutrition and vitamin B3.) Life became a nightmare of apparently "imaginary condition".

1974: "Cured of long-endured illness. Felt as if life had begun again."

Irene passed away in February 1991.

Talk to your doctor

You're not feeling well, so you go to see your doctor.

Scenario One: You say, "I seem to be hungry constantly and if I don't eat on time, I get dizzy and really irritable". Your doctor says "Do you instantly feel better when you eat?" When you nod, she says, "Maybe your blood sugar is dropping too much. Let's do some tests and explore this a bit."

Scenario Two: You say, "I think I may have hypoglycemia". Your doctor says, "OK, lets have a look at how you are feeling and check all of the possibilities".

These are ideal situations, and maybe you are one of the lucky people whose doctor understands hypoglycemia in non-diabetics, or at least is open-minded enough to explore the possibility. The doctor will probably refer you to a nutritionist or give you some diet guidelines. He may still order additional tests to ensure that there aren't other underlying problems, but you will feel confident that you are on the road to recovery.

Unfortunately, most people don't have an experience that positive. More often, your doctor won't know about hypoglycemia, outside of diabetes, anyway. And if he has heard of it, chances are good that he thinks it is a fad problem, and that those who think they have hypoglycemia are really hypochondriacs or are suffering from heart murmur, depression or panic attacks.

Most hypoglycemics see many doctors and endure many tests before finding out that what they really need is a change in diet. In the meantime, they have tried many different treatments including thyroid drugs and anti-depressants. Even your suggestion that your problems might stem from low blood sugar is no guarantee that your doctor will progress more quickly to testing that will confirm hypoglycemia.

Keep in mind that a good doctor will want to check all of the possibilities, and will want to ensure that your blood sugar fluctuations aren't caused by something life threatening. Remember, your doctor is concerned with making a *correct* diagnosis, not a quick one.

Think of it this way. Suppose you took your misbehaving car to a mechanic. You were pretty sure that the problem was the spark plugs, so the mechanic replaced the spark plugs and that's all. If your car was to break down the very next week because the transmission stopped working, you would be upset, wouldn't you? After the inconvenience of having your car in the shop, he didn't find all of the problems and you had to take it in again. If he had checked your car out more thoroughly the first time, chances are that you wouldn't have had to come back again so soon.

Suppose you went to your doctor and said, "I think I have hypoglycemia." After a few questions, the doctor agrees and sends you to a nutritionist. This sounds great, but what if there is another problem that is contributing to your hypoglycemia? As an example, hypoglycemia symptoms can be exacerbated by poor thyroid function, and hypothyroid can be very successfully treated with hormones. Treating this problem will make your hypoglycemia much easier to deal with.

Another thing to consider is that if you have been hypoglycemic for a long time, insulin resistance may already be causing additional problems—high blood pressure, for example. This is very important information, and may affect your treatment.

Because hypoglycemia is not a disease in itself, it is very difficult to separate causes from effects. Is hypoglycemia causing all your problems, or is something else causing your hypoglycemia? Additional testing may be very important in sorting it all out. Allergies and other medical conditions complicate the picture as well. How hypoglycemia is linked to a series of other conditions was explored in the previous chapter—it doesn't often appear in isolation.

Why don't doctors talk about hypoglycemia?

Hypoglycemia causes a strange group of symptoms that could stem from many other conditions, including psychological ones. In addition, the only and best treatment for hypoglycemia is a change in diet. Medical school is a high pressure, high workload place to be, and one of the main reasons is the huge volume of information that has to be learned and applied. This is not a place for the weak or timid!

There are new diseases and viruses demanding to be added to the curriculum, and it is easy to imagine that they simply run out of time for subjects considered "basic" or "common sense" like diet. After all, in North America, the US and Canadian Food Guides tell us what we should be eating. We hardly need a doctor for that, do we?

Besides, there are so many conditions for which the diagnosis and treatment are very complex and mistakes can be life threatening. Something as simple as diet doesn't need much attention. Does it?

What did my doctor learn about hypoglycemia?

When doctors learn about hypoglycemia, they learn that it is a condition caused by a mismatch of food, exercise and insulin in diabetics. They learn that this can be life threatening and that proper and immediate treatment is necessary. Many have learned that hypoglycemia is very rare in people without diabetes. This is the last thing they learn to look for in someone who is not diabetic, unless, of course, they suspect insulin abuse or a pancreatic tumor.

Doctors who read to keep up with advances in medical knowledge, and many of them do, may have heard about hypoglycemia in non-diabetics. If they happen to explore further, though, most of the medical literature will tell them that hypoglycemia in non-diabetics is one of the new "fad diseases" that has captured the attention of the masses. It will re-assert and confirm to your doctor that hypoglycemia is very rare in non-diabetics. She will leave testing for hypoglycemia until after she has checked for all of the "more likely" possibilities or she may never do the testing at all.

Diet as cause

Neglecting to teach medical students the effects of diet is an unfortunate omission. The human body is a system like many others, both natural and manufactured, and what goes in affects not only what goes out, but also how well it operates.

Consider other professions:

If your car is running poorly, one of the first questions your mechanic will ask is "What kind of fuel are you using?"

If the shrubbery in your yard is going brown, the nursery will ask "How much water is it getting, and are you feeding it?"

If your dog or your horse is seen by the vet for anything from digestive problems to skin rashes or dull coat, the first thing the vet will check is his diet.

The situation is better for babies and children than it is for adults. I remember taking my baby daughter to our doctor for a routine check-up and the doctor noticed that her skin color was off. "Has she been eating a lot of carrots?" (I guess she did like carrots a bit too much!)

In adult humans, it's a different story altogether.

"I have a rash"—use this cream.

"I have diarrhea"—try this medication.

"I'm often dizzy"—take this drug.

All of these conditions (and lots of others) can be caused by your diet. I don't know about you, but I have never had a doctor ask about my diet.

This is partly our own fault, too. We are all impatient for the quick fix and doctors have figured out how to keep us happy. They know that if they tell us to cut out the sweets to feel better or to lose weight, we leave the office feeling low. Perhaps we feel that we are being blamed for the problem. Besides, the cure is *difficult*. Most important of all, we won't feel better by tomorrow!

If instead, they hand us a prescription, we leave happy. We have something immediate we can do, and we can be pretty sure we will be feeling better soon.

Is it any wonder that our doctors are quick to hand out prescriptions rather than tell us to stop eating desserts? It's time we take some responsibility for our own "cures". It's time to start asking what else *we* could be doing, and whether there are bad habits *we* could change.

How can I talk to my doctor about hypoglycemia?

Your doctor is a highly trained professional and is used to knowing more about your body and how it operates than you do. She is comfortable with this situation and may be surprised, and even dismayed, when you come in with a ready made self-diagnosis—hypoglycemia. And if your doctor has already heard all about this "fad", she may be suspicious of it as well.

Remember, your doctor is only human. Highly educated and highly intelligent, but still human. This means that she might also be uncomfortable if you seem to be encroaching on her area of expertise.

When you go, go armed with all the facts. It will be much easier for her to take you seriously if you have done your homework. Take your food journal, complete with symptoms. If you have been taking blood sugar readings, have them with you. If your food journal includes blood sugar readings that correspond to the symptoms you experienced, better yet.

In preparing for your visit to your doctor, consider this list of tips. It was written by Dr. Mendosa for diabetics, but it applies equally well for hypoglycemics. It was posted on his website at the time of this writing (www.mendosa.com):

▌ *Sit down and think about your upcoming visit: the reason for the visit and any change in your diabetes or other illnesses you may have had since the last time you saw the doctor.*

▌ *If you have particular symptoms to report, think about what time of day they happen, how long they last, whether they have been getting worse or better, and whether or not they interfere with your daily activities.*

▌ *Prepare a list of questions and concerns beforehand (it's not as easy to think when you're on that exam table!). Prioritize your list so that you make sure to get your most pressing concerns addressed.*

▌ *Provide a complete list of medications (prescription and over-the-counter), including any pain relievers, vitamins, supplements and herbs you are taking or have taken recently.*

▌ *Research (online, at the library, or through your insurance company) new treatments or medications for diabetes that you may want to discuss with your doctor.*

▌ *Make notes of what the doctor says. You can do this in the exam room or in the waiting room after your appointment. Be sure that you know what the doctor said and that you understand any medical terms he or she used. If not, ask for an explanation before you leave.*

If you have trouble talking to your doctor and remembering what you wanted to ask, this should help. And if you ever have trouble remembering your doctor's explanations or advice, you may find this list of tips very useful.

If your doctor isn't familiar with testing for hypoglycemia and how to interpret the results, you might consider taking some doctor friendly information with you. One book I found very useful is *Hypoglycemia: The Disease Your Doctor Won't Treat* by Jeraldine Saunders and Dr. Harvey M. Ross.

This is a very useful resource because it describes the GTT procedure in detail and includes graphics showing how to read the results for hypoglycemia. Because of his medical degree, Dr. Ross's description is more likely to be accepted by your doctor.

If, in spite of your best efforts, your doctor is unable or unwilling to help, consider enlisting the help of a holistic doctor. Holistic doctors are committed to treating the "whole you", and not just your body. This means that they work with you on all aspects of your life, including your nutrition.

Holistic doctors

It is more important to know what sort of patient has the disease than what sort of disease the patient has.—Sir William Osler

Holistic doctors are interested in who you are and how you live. They want to know how you feel and how your lifestyle affects your health. A holistic doctor will probably talk (and listen) a lot more than the doctors you have become used to, and may ask you to fill in a comprehensive questionnaire during your first visit. And rest assured, a holistic doctor will ask you about your diet!

Keep in mind that just because a doctor might incorporate alternative therapies in her practice, that doesn't mean that she is a holistic doctor. Conversely, a so-called "traditional" doctor may practice medicine in a holistic way.

An environment in which your doctor treats you as a person rather than as a disease is an ideal environment for you to learn to manage your hypoglycemia. In the search for a good holistic doctor, though, it is still "buyer beware", and you will have to choose carefully. The American Holistic Medical Association offers the following very useful advice for choosing a holistic practitioner. (see Table 4)

In addition to this list, I would advise: *Make sure that this practitioner has a medical degree.*

The American Holistic Medical Association has a mandate *"to support practitioners in their evolving personal and professional development as healers and to educate physicians about holistic medicine"*. Members include Medical Doctors (MD's), Doctors of Osteopathy and medical students. In addition to promoting education of their members and research in Alternative Medicine, the AHMA also operates an on-line physician referral service to help you find a holistic doctor in your area. You can find the AMHA website at www.holisticmedicine.org.

The American Board of Holistic Medicine runs regular testing for doctors wishing to become certified in holistic medicine, and the general testing includes sections on Physical (environmental medicine, exercise medicine and nutritional medicine); Mental (Psychological Medicine, Psychoneuroimmunolgy, Relaxation and Voluntary Controls); and Spiritual/Social Health. There are also six specialized sections: Biomolecular Medicine, Botanical Medicine, Energy Medicine, Ethnomedicine, Homeopathic Medicine and Manual Medicine.

Table 4: Choosing a Holistic Practitioner

How to Choose a Holistic Practitioner

Your first responsibility as a patient/client is to select a practitioner who will join your "team" to support you in obtaining and maintaining optimum health for your body, mind, emotions and spirit. While most holistic practitioners use modalities that are currently labeled "alternative medicine", the interests and practices of our members vary widely. Thus, one person might work primarily with nutrition and herbs, while another might look mainly at the spiritual aspects of health and disease. Other areas of interest include spinal manipulation and bodywork, "energy medicine", mind-body medicine, acupuncture and stress management. It is important to remember that there are many different definitions of holistic medicine. When choosing a practitioner, make sure that individual has the same type of philosophy and uses the treatment modalities you are seeking.

The following considerations are offered as a guide to help you find a practitioner with whom you are comfortable. Optimum health is more likely to be present when you work with someone who is supportive of your efforts to be in charge of your life. Some of the criteria may not apply to all situations.

1. ***Does this practitioner have healthy professional relationships with others?*** *How did you hear about this practitioner? A personal referral is often more powerful than a professional referral. What do friends and other professionals say about this person? How does he/she feel about second opinions or your interest in alternative health care therapies/treatments? What technical certifications, professional organizations or hospital affiliations does this practitioner have?*

Table 4: (cont.)

2. *How do YOU respond to this practitioner's office and staff?* This environment reveals his/her attitudes and beliefs. Do you feel comfortable and cared for when you call or visit the office? Does the ambiance enhance that comfort? Does the staff further your sense of well being? Are educational handouts available in the office or waiting room? Is your appointment time honored or do you have to wait?

3. *Do you feel like a valued person working as a partner with this practitioner?* Healing is enhanced by a healthy relationship between patient/client and practitioner. Do you feel this practitioner is there for you? Do you feel trust and confidence? Does he/she seem to care about you, take your medical history personally and show an interest in your family, lifestyle and diet? Are you told about various treatment options? Does each of you recognize that you need the other? Is the practitioner accessible? Are you able to discuss the financial aspects of your care openly and comfortably? Positive answers to these questions are evidence of your rightful place as a co-creator of this healing partnership.

4. *Is your personal dignity respected?* Any examination or interaction should be respectful of your personal dignity.

5. *Does this practitioner honor your anxieties and fears?* Is this practitioner sensitive enough to place him/herself in your position regarding fears and anxieties about an illness or proposed treatment?

6. *What is the state of this practitioner's health?* Does he/she appear to have a healthy lifestyle? Signs of overweight, overwork, smoking or drinking may indicate that he/she does not take care of him/herself. You

Table 4: (cont.)

> will probably do best with a team member who is just as committed to good health as you are. The Biblical statement, "Physician, heal thyself", is paramount in a health-filled relationship.

7. *Are you allowed time between diagnosis and treatment?* Does this practitioner allow you the time to collect the educational and personal resources that you need to make a well-informed decision?

8. *Are you treated as if this is an important, ongoing relationship?* Are you notified of test results within a reasonable period of time? Are follow-up visits scheduled after treatment? Is there discussion of future health goals and not just the immediate matter at hand?

9. *Do you feel unconditionally accepted by this practitioner?* Unconditional acceptance allows you to get well in your unique way. Do you feel that you are accepted no matter what develops, no matter what decisions you make? Can the practitioner approach your care with an open mind, rather than with a predetermined treatment plan? Would the practitioner offer to a member of his/her own family the same carefully chosen advice that he/she has offered to you?

10. *Would you send the person most dear to you to this practitioner?* Do you have such a strong feeling of caring, confidence and trust in this practitioner that you would send to him/her, with no misgivings, the person who is dearest to you? If so, then you have found that special person to be on your health team.

Source: Taken from the American Holistic Medical Association website: holisticmedicine.org with permission.

I reproduce the list here to illustrate the breadth of the knowledge required for certification in Holistic Medicine by the American Board of Holistic Medicine.

That said, just because some holistic practitioners are qualified in this way doesn't mean that every person who hangs out a "Holistic" shingle is. Check credentials. You should at least make sure that your holistic doctor has a medical degree.

In Canada, organizations with a holistic focus include the Canadian Complementary Medical Association and the Canadian Holistic Medical Association. The CCMA was founded in 1996 to *"encourage education of physicians and public, complementary medical research and support for doctors practising complementary medical therapies"*. The physician directory was not yet in service at the time of this writing, but a spokesperson for the association says that it will be in service soon. (www.ccmadoctors.ca)

The Canadian Holistic Medical Association was founded in 1977 by Dr. Edward Leyton of Kingston, Ontario and defines Holistic Medicine as *"a system of health care which fosters a cooperative relationship among all those involved, leading towards optimal attainment of the physical, mental, emotional, social and spiritual aspects of health"*. (www3.sympatico.ca/holodoc/)

Remember, no matter who you see for help, you are still in charge, and it is up to you to find a suitable doctor. It is also up to you to help work out a treatment plan that you can commit to. Your willingness to take responsibility for your own health is the most important component of any treatment no matter what medical professionals you see.

Whether or not you are successful in finding a doctor who can help, you will probably still need help from a nutrition professional. This is where dietitians and nutritionists come in.

Dietitians and nutritionists

If you have trouble finding a holistic doctor in your area, a dietician may be the most knowledgeable professional you will have access to.

Becoming a dietitian requires a four-year university degree, and candidates learn everything from what constitutes a good exercise program to how to talk to people about nutrition and how to manage a large scale, institutional kitchen. In addition to the classroom training, dietitians get hands on experience through a job assignment ranging in length from 20-35 weeks.

North American dietitians are certified by the Dietitians of Canada or the American Dietetic Association. The Manual of Dietetics is managed jointly by the two organizations, so the requirements and expectations in the two countries is compatible and overlaps as well. In Canada, you can tell a registered dietitian by his or her credentials—only registered dietitians are permitted to use the letters RD, RDN, PDt or RDt (in Quebec, the French equivalent Dt.P.). In the USA, the legal designations are RD, DTR, CSP (Pediatric Nutrition) and CSR (Specialist for Renal Nutrition). The designation "dietitian" is protected by law and can only be used by people with a dietetics degree from an accredited university, related ethics training and at least one year of experience in the field.

It surprised me to learn that the Dietitians' education standards didn't explicitly mention the treatment of hypoglycemia. In fact, the Dietitians of Canada representative for Education Standards seemed surprised about this too. She assured me that it was "definitely covered" in the approved curriculum for professional dietitians. "Reactive Hypoglycemia" did appear in the Table of Contents of the Manual of Dietetics.

In recent years, dietitians have been moving from the institutional settings they are most known for (hospitals and seniors homes) to private practice. In private practice, dieticians often list themselves as *nutritionists*.

Nutritionist is not a protected designation, so not every nutritionist you meet will have a university degree in dietetics. In Canada, dietitians are also provincially registered, and in America, forty-six states register dietitians, so if you have doubts, check with your state or provincial regulator. For American Dietitian information, visit www.eatright.org. A contact for information is listed for each state. The site also includes a "dietitian finder" to help you locate a registered professional in your neighborhood. The Dieticians of Canada website, www.dietitians.ca, also offers help in finding a registered dietitian, and its information pages and FAQ (Frequently Asked Questions) are interesting and informative.

This is not to say that nutritionists without degrees are necessarily bad, but it is important to know the educational background and credentials of anyone you are trusting with your health.

A dietitian/nutritionist will help you with your diet by educating you on the best ways to get a "balanced" diet that includes the right proportion of carbohydrates, proteins and fats. She will be able to recommend nutritional supplements and a good place to buy high quality products. She may also make suggestions on how you can add to or change your exercise regimen for optimum improvement.

When you meet dietitians or nutritionists, don't be shy. Ask to see their credentials, ask where they studied and most important, ask how they treat hypoglycemia. If you are uncomfortable with any of their answers, leave. You won't have trouble locating others; the American Dietetic Association alone has 70,000 members.

Chapter 11

Continuing the journey

■ ■ ■ ■ *After years of craving sugar and sweets all the time, in May of 2002, I stopped eating sugar.*

After years of headaches, depression, weight gain (and loss); after years of wondering why I didn't feel up to getting through the day; after years of wondering why I just didn't seem to living up to my potential; after years of wishing I could actually concentrate on something, I finally started to work on myself. I started with exercise by going to the gym twice a week. I began to feel better and I became stronger, but I didn't lose any weight and I still didn't have any energy. I finally decided that it was time to learn about hypoglycemia.

I had first heard about hypoglycemia years earlier and as I visited hypoglycemia web sites, I could see that all the symptoms matched mine. And I began to see a disturbing trend. Almost every web site's first message was "Stop eating sugar." Now that was drastic. I couldn't imagine life without cookies.

After a couple of months of talking myself into it, I finally decided to take the plunge and give up sugar.

To get help adjusting to the changes and to find out about supplements I should be taking, I started seeing Dr. Todd Norton, a nutritionist recommended by a friend. On my first visit, he had me fill out a comprehensive survey, and twigged on my report of longstanding eczema on my hands. He confirmed that my body was definitely having trouble dealing with sugar, but he decided that I should also give up wheat, corn, caffeine and all dairy foods.

What a shock to my system.

It wasn't easy, and as in many of the stories you've read, I felt worse before I felt better. I craved sugar intensely and I was extremely irritable. I felt lost. I didn't know what to eat, and I couldn't concentrate on anything. I was already working on this book, but I certainly wasn't getting much done! But by the end of the month (late June), my eczema was gone, and I found that dairy was OK, but wheat and corn were not. (Movies without popcorn? No way!)

In early July, we flew across Canada for a 50th wedding anniversary party. I found that there were new hurdles. What can I eat at the airport? What can I eat on the plane? How can I avoid sugar, alcohol and wheat at a party?

The party was a real challenge. The tables were laden with food, little sandwiches, sweet desserts and champagne. Not one thing that I could put in my mouth.

Well, I got through that party and the days that followed, but not without mistakes and getting home meant working hard at my routine once again.

By the time I got to August, I suddenly realized that I wasn't coughing. This was significant because I had been coughing my way through the summers for at least five years. I had been told that it was due to dust and dog allergies and I had been using an inhaler to control the coughing. I still had the dog, and I hadn't been cleaning any more than I ever did, but I wasn't coughing.

Because I eliminated sugar, wheat and corn at the same time, it is impossible to be sure how much credit I should give each of these changes for the amazing improvements I have experienced in my health, but it doesn't matter much—I feel so much better in every way. I was joking the other day that I thought I must have de-aged ten years!

By September of 2002, all of my symptoms were subsiding and my concentration was improving, but I still hadn't completely given up caffeine. I was still seeing Dr. Norton, and at every appointment he reminded me that I really needed to give up caffeine. This was my toughest challenge. Caffeine helped me to feel happy and alert, and although I was only drinking about a half a diet cola per day (from four each day), I was still refusing to give it up completely.

In September, I finally kicked the caffeine habit. It was still hard, but I was able to do it because I was feeling better in so many ways.

Within weeks, I found that my sleep was improving. I have never slept well my whole life, and I was now sleeping through the night. Sleeping better is probably the biggest and most important change I've experienced since changing my diet.

By late fall, I had more energy than I had ever had. I always thought that I was just naturally a low-energy person. But now I was busy, active and mentally alert from 6:00 am through to 9:00 pm. Seemed like a miracle!

Another surprising side effect was that I was losing weight. I have been trying to slim down on and off for years, but with no success. Now the fat was simply melting away. I was so afraid of jinxing it by becoming obsessed with tracking it, but for the first time, I wasn't hungry or irritable and I was continuing to lose. By the beginning of December, I had lost 25 pounds. I haven't looked so good in years.

Christmas brought the usual challenges and I met each as it came, although I ate some foods I shouldn't have. I paid for every lapse with a return of symptoms and I learned from my mistakes. My parents visited us for a week over the holidays. Their visits have always been high stress events for me, but this time I was able to relax, and for the first time in over 20 years, the tension didn't consume me and ruin our visit.

Three years later, I am still dealing with the challenges, and chocolate is the biggest one for me. I still occasionally break that cardinal rule (sugar and caffeine), but now I know that I will be able to get it under control again.

I am happier than I have ever been. I am optimistic and energetic. I have great hope for the future and I know it will only get better. I am still a few pounds over my ideal weight, but I simply refuse to worry about it. If it comes off, it does. And if it doesn't, I am healthier than ever before and that is the best gift I have ever given myself!

ANITA FLEGG

You can do it

Hypoglycemia is a daunting condition that requires work to treat, especially when it hides in a crowd of linked conditions like those listed in Chapter 9. There is hope, though. As you read the personal stories that introduced each chapter, you met some people struggling with hypoglycemia. They have not fully gained control of their symptoms, but they all have hope that better days are coming. You also met hypoglycemics who are already living very full, very productive lives. This is what you can aspire to. It may not be easy, but you can improve how you feel and how well you function. You can gain a measure of control by changing and improving the way you take care of yourself. I challenge you to get going today by starting the Workbook in the next section of this book.

You have what it takes. You can make your life and your health better. Don't wait. Start on the workbook in the next section now. It's never too late to improve the rest of your life.

Go for it!

Getting control of your Hypoglycemia Step by Step

You've read the book and you are starting to think that you probably have hypoglycemia. What to do next? This workbook is the answer.

First, you will complete a Symptoms Checklist that will help you to find out whether or not you have hypoglycemia. The rest of this workbook will guide you through the Steps needed to get your blood sugar—and your symptoms—under control.

Work through each of the Steps in the order given, but take as long as you need for each one. There is no right or wrong time frame for working your way through the workbook. You can start each Step when you are ready.

The most important piece of advice I can give you as you begin is to be patient with yourself. The effects of years of eating sugar and refined foods cannot be reversed overnight. It will take some time and effort and you will need to adjust to new eating habits and new shopping habits. But rest assured, it will be worth it. You will feel better!

Congratulations on making a start—you can improve your health and your life!

Hypoglycemia Workbook

Step 1 — Symptom Checklist

The first Step is to figure out if your health problems could be caused by hypoglycemia. Use this Symptoms Checklist to find out.

This Checklist cannot substitute for the advice of your doctor, but you can take it to your next appointment and use it when you talk to him or her about hypoglycemia. This Checklist can also be useful as a starting point when talking to your nutritionist.

As you go through this workbook, you will use this checklist as a baseline of your current symptoms. As you work through the Steps you will redo the Symptom checklist and you will be able to see how your symptoms improve.

For all of the symptoms that affect you, mark their frequency and severity using the following scale.

Frequency
- *Daily* – The symptom occurs at least once every day.
- *Weekly* – The symptom occurs at least once every week. Select Weekly if you have the symptom more than once a week, but not on a daily basis.
- *Monthly* – The symptom occurs only occasionally.

Severity
- *Mild* – You notice the symptom, but it does not impact your activities. For example, if you have a headache that does not stop you from working or completing an activity, it's a mild symptom.
- *Moderate* – The symptom has some impact on your activities, but you are still able to function reasonably normally.
- *Severe* – The symptom interferes with your day. You either have to change activities or delay an activity until the symptom subsides.

Symptom Checklist

	Frequency			Severity		
	Daily	Weekly	Monthly	Mild	Moderate	Severe
My heart races	❏	❏	❏	❏	❏	❏
I am irritable before eating (better after I eat)	❏	❏	❏	❏	❏	❏
I tremble or feel shaky	❏	❏	❏	❏	❏	❏
I suddenly start sweating	❏	❏	❏	❏	❏	❏
I feel clammy all over	❏	❏	❏	❏	❏	❏
I feel like I am trembling inside	❏	❏	❏	❏	❏	❏
I feel nauseous	❏	❏	❏	❏	❏	❏
My hands and feet are cold	❏	❏	❏	❏	❏	❏
I am constantly hungry	❏	❏	❏	❏	❏	❏
I feel mentally "cloudy"	❏	❏	❏	❏	❏	❏
My pupils are dilated	❏	❏	❏	❏	❏	❏
I feel faint	❏	❏	❏	❏	❏	❏
I feel apprehensive	❏	❏	❏	❏	❏	❏
I am tired	❏	❏	❏	❏	❏	❏
I have headaches or migraines	❏	❏	❏	❏	❏	❏
I feel dizzy	❏	❏	❏	❏	❏	❏
I have blurred or double vision	❏	❏	❏	❏	❏	❏
I have insomnia or other sleep problems	❏	❏	❏	❏	❏	❏
I have difficulty concentrating	❏	❏	❏	❏	❏	❏
My mood changes suddenly	❏	❏	❏	❏	❏	❏
I am anxious or nervous	❏	❏	❏	❏	❏	❏
I have outbursts of temper	❏	❏	❏	❏	❏	❏
I feel disoriented	❏	❏	❏	❏	❏	❏
I have trouble making decisions	❏	❏	❏	❏	❏	❏
I am forgetful	❏	❏	❏	❏	❏	❏
	Always	Often	Some-times	Never		
My symptoms disappear after I eat ...	❏	❏	❏	❏		

Hypoglycemia Workbook

If you have many of these symptoms, it is very possible that you have hypoglycemia. If the symptoms seem to improve after you eat, it is even more likely that the problem is hypoglycemia.

If you have more than 5 of these symptoms or if any of them are **Severe**, please see your doctor.

If you have some of these symptoms every day or some of these symptoms stop you from functioning normally, following the Steps in this workbook will help you experience fewer symptoms less often.

After you have spent a few weeks working through the diet changes suggested in the following Steps, you will do the survey again so that you can compare how you feel to how you felt when you started.

If you think you have hypoglycemia, proceed to Step 2 and start on the road to improved health!

> Try adding a multivitamin with minerals, Vitamin C and Chromium to help stabilize your blood sugar.

Step 2 — Track your eating habits and your symptoms with a Food Journal

In this Step, you will keep a food journal for at least a week. This journal will help you find the links between what you eat and how you feel. Eat as you normally would and track how you feel. You may be surprised at what you find.

After a week or two of journaling:

▪ You will have a better idea of how often your symptoms are actually appearing.

▪ You will learn what times of day your symptoms most often appear.

▪ You will start to notice trends, for example, the times of the day you are most hungry and what you most often do to relieve your symptoms.

▪ You will notice if there are any particular foods that always cause symptoms.

▪ You will notice when you feel your best.

Your Journal, along with the Symptoms Checklist you completed in Step 1 will be a good tool to take to your doctor or nutritionist because it will tell them exactly how you are doing.

Here's how to keep your Food Journal

To get started, copy the sample journal on the next page or download it from www.theOtherSugarDisease.com. Re-read pages 121-125 for more about keeping a Food Journal.

1. Write in the date.
2. For everything you put into your mouth, write down what you ate and how much and the time you ate it.
3. Write down how you felt just before you ate and again after you ate. Pay attention to your body and if you start to feel better or if you start to have unpleasant symptoms, write these in the "How do I feel" column along with the time the feeling started.

Use as much space as you need to record how you are feeling before and after you eat.

Keep your Journal handy all the time. Take it to work with you and when you are at home, keep it on the fridge with a magnet. Make sure you have extra copies of the blank journal page so that you are always ready for the next snack or the next note.

Keep your food journal for at least a week—2 or 3 weeks will be even better. When you think you have enough eating history to allow you to see some trends, proceed to Step 3.

Pick one meeting this week and decide not to eat a donut. Treat yourself to some nuts or a piece of cheese before or after the meeting (or both).

Food Journal

Date	Time	Food/Amount	How do I feel?

Hypoglycemia Workbook

Step 3 — Interpret your Food Journal

Your Symptom Checklist and Food Journal are great tools for getting a better understanding of your body and how it reacts to various foods. You will also start to understand how often you need to eat to feel well.

You can interpret your completed Food Journal by writing down the answers to these questions.

▌ How often are you eating now? Are you eating constantly or are you forgetting to eat? Are you just eating 3 meals per day?

_____

_____

_____

_____

_____

▌ How do you generally feel just before eating? Is this the same every day?

_____

_____

_____

_____

_____

▌ When you are experiencing symptoms, what do you usually do? Do you eat, and if so, what do you eat? Is it usually something sweet?

_____

_____

_____

_____

_____

▌ What times of the day are you most likely to have symptoms? For instance, do you always feel bad at 11:00am? Or when you first get up in the morning?

_____

_____

_____

_____

_____

▮ When reading the symptoms you recorded on the chart, look at the foods you ate that day. Do these symptoms always appear when you eat those foods?

_____

_____

_____

_____

_____

To give you an idea of what to look for: When I started journaling, I found that I lost concentration at work at about 10:00am and again at about 3:00pm. It was always at these times that I would go looking for a cookie, a muffin or a chocolate bar. I hated going to meetings that were scheduled for just before lunch because I really couldn't listen properly. I always felt better right after eating.

I found that I started to lose concentration or got a headache or got really hungry within 2 hours of eating. I craved sweets pretty much all of the time.

I also noticed that I was having headaches every day, whether I was working or not. And I noticed that I got really bad headaches within 10 minutes of having the fruit drink that I bought for the kids' lunches.

This is the kind of information that is really valuable when understanding how to make the changes that you will need to make to reduce your symptoms. You will use this information in later Steps.

Record any additional observations here:

_____

_____

_____

_____

_____

_____

_____

_____

_____

_____

_____

Instead of coffee in the late afternoon, have water with lemon or perhaps herbal tea. Have a protein snack with it, and after a few days, you probably won't even miss it.

Hypoglycemia Workbook

Step 4 — Change When and What you eat

Calculate your optimum Eating Cycle

You can minimize the symptoms of hypoglycemia by eating at regular intervals and by finding the Eating Cycle that works for you. Your Eating Cycle is the maximum amount of time you should allow yourself to go without eating during the day.

1. Review your Food Journal. Look for the interval of time between when you ate and when you experienced symptoms.

2. The minimum time between eating and symptoms is

   _____.

3. Subtract 30 minutes from your minimum time. The result is _____.

   This number is your Eating Cycle.

Change your eating habits so that you eat more small meals. The times between your meals and snacks should not exceed your Eating Cycle.

For example, if your Food Journal shows that you get headaches or other symptoms 3 hours after you eat, then the calculation above would give an Eating Cycle of 2.5 hours. In other words, you need to eat every 2.5 hours. If you eat breakfast at 8:00am, then you need a snack at 10:30am, lunch at 1:00pm, another snack at 3:30pm, supper at 6:00pm and a snack at 8:30pm.

Eat at the scheduled time even if you do not feel hungry. If you know you will be away from home, be sure to take a snack with you. If you know you won't be able to eat at the proper time, eat early to avoid the onset of symptoms.

What to eat

Now you know how often to eat. It may seem like a lot and you may wonder what on earth you will eat!

Plan to follow these new rules for at least two weeks. At the same time, stick with your Food Journal. This will help you see if your symptoms are improving.

Here are the three most important rules:

❶ Eat 6-8 times each day according to the calculation you just did above.

❷ Eat protein in every meal and snack. Some examples of protein food:

meat	cheese	fish	lentils
seeds	eggs	yogurt	tofu

nuts (almonds, walnuts, pistachios…)

❸ Eat only high fiber carbohydrates. That means eating lots of vegetables, and having them raw as often as possible. It also means eliminating refined foods like white bread and white rice.

After 2 to 3 weeks of following the new rules, proceed to Step 5.

Choose to skip one cigarette break each day and treat yourself to a protein snack instead.

Step 5 — Reduce your sugar intake

If you have hypoglycemia, this means that you have difficulty metabolizing sugar, so one of the keys to feeling better is to reduce your sugar intake. Your ultimate target is to eliminate most or all of the sugar from your diet.

You might be surprised to hear just how much sugar there is in many of the foods we eat regularly. Here is a list I found at www.cspinet.org/reports/sugar/popsugar.html.

FOOD	TSP Sugar
Snickers bar, 2.1 oz.	5 ¾
Lowfat fruit-flavored yogurt, 8 oz.	7
*Burger King Cini-minis w/icing,** 4.7 oz.	9 ½
Pepsi, 12 oz.	10 ¼
Pancake syrup, ¼ cup	10 ¼
*McDonald's Vanilla Shake,** 20 oz.	12
*Cinnabon,** 7 ½ oz.	12 ¼
Sunkist Orange Soda, 12 oz.	13
*McDonald's McFlurry with Butterfingers,** 10 oz.	13 ¾
Strawberry Passion Awareness Fruitopia, 20 oz.	17 ¾
Dairy Queen Mr. Misty Slush,** 32 oz.	28

Sources: Manufacturers, USDA, *CSPI analyses* and/or estimates.

Center for Science in the Public Interest, August, 1999

* These products trademarks are the property of their respective companies.

If you are currently eating a lot of sugar every day, you may want to step down your sugar intake over several weeks instead of going "cold turkey". Try cutting your sugar intake in half. Once your system adjusts to this, step down by cutting your sugar intake in half again. Allow your body to adjust again, and then cut the intake in half again. Continue doing this until your sugar intake is low enough that you can cut out sugar altogether.

You can reduce your sugar intake by reducing or cutting out:

- Sugar in your coffee and tea (cut the sugar in half; you'll find that you get used to it very quickly)
- Sugary desserts (have half a piece of cake or half a scoop of ice cream)
- Soft drinks (if you usually have 2 per day, cut back to 1 per day, for example)
- Fruit drinks and fruit juice (substitute whole fruit, or mix with water)
- Energy drinks (replace with water)
- Chocolate bars, candy (cut back to half as much as you would usually have)
- Snack foods such as muffins, doughnuts, cookies, granola bars (cut back to half servings)
- Sugar coated or frosted breakfast cereals (switch to non-sugared cereals or cut the sugar you add in half)

Write down some ways you will cut down on the amount of sugar you eat:

_____

_____

_____

_____

_____

Hypoglycemia Workbook

Whether you reduce your sugar intake slowly or all at once, you may experience strong cravings that make it very difficult to stick to your plan. Here are some things you can try to ease the cravings and help you think about other things.

- Eat a protein snack
- Go for a walk
- Work on your hobby
- Call a friend
- Go to the gym for a workout
- Take your children to the park
- Put your favorite music on the stereo and dance around the living room
- Write a list of all the things you will be better able to do once your hypoglycemia symptoms have improved.

If you are the type to do all or nothing and you plan to eliminate sugar cold turkey, keep in mind that your symptoms may get quite a bit worse before they get better. If you go cold turkey, it won't be very useful to keep a Food Journal during the weeks of your sugar "withdrawal". Wait 3-4 weeks before beginning to journal again.

Keep the cookies/chips/soft drinks out of your grocery cart this week. When the kids go looking for a snack, remind them how good yogurt and fresh fruit is or give them a small bowl of trail mix to eat while they do their homework.

Make your own list of things that you will do to distract yourself when the sugar cravings hit.

_____

_____

_____

_____

_____

_____

_____

_____

Try to avoid substituting artificial sweeteners such as Splenda™, Aspartame™ or the herb stevia. For some people, even the sweet taste can trigger an insulin response that can cause low blood sugar symptoms. If you must use a sweetener occasionally, go with stevia; it is the least likely to have an effect on your blood sugar.

Once you have cut out sugar and your cravings have subsided, you will know that the worst has passed and your health will continue to improve. You may already be noticing that your symptoms are less frequent or less severe.

Continue to Step 6 and complete the Symptom Checklist again to check your progress.

Hypoglycemia Workbook

Step 6 — Still having symptoms?

Fill in the Symptom Checklist again. This is an important step because it will help you see how far you have already come.

Compare this checklist to the one you completed in Step 1.

As you look at your Symptoms Checklist from Step 1, pick out the symptoms that you marked as happening *Daily*. Have any of them moved to the *Weekly* or even the *Monthly* column?

Have any of the Symptoms that you originally rated as *Severe* become *Moderate* or *Mild*? Even if you still rated some of your symptoms as Severe and they are still happening *Daily*, have you noticed some improvement?

Symptom Checklist

	Frequency			Severity		
	Daily	Weekly	Monthly	Mild	Moderate	Severe
My heart races	❑	❑	❑	❑	❑	❑
I am irritable before eating (better after I eat)	❑	❑	❑	❑	❑	❑
I tremble or feel shaky	❑	❑	❑	❑	❑	❑
I suddenly start sweating	❑	❑	❑	❑	❑	❑
I feel clammy all over	❑	❑	❑	❑	❑	❑
I feel like I am trembling inside	❑	❑	❑	❑	❑	❑
I feel nauseous	❑	❑	❑	❑	❑	❑
My hands and feet are cold	❑	❑	❑	❑	❑	❑
I am constantly hungry	❑	❑	❑	❑	❑	❑
I feel mentally "cloudy"	❑	❑	❑	❑	❑	❑
My pupils are dilated	❑	❑	❑	❑	❑	❑
I feel faint	❑	❑	❑	❑	❑	❑
I feel apprehensive	❑	❑	❑	❑	❑	❑
I am tired	❑	❑	❑	❑	❑	❑
I have headaches or migraines	❑	❑	❑	❑	❑	❑
I feel dizzy	❑	❑	❑	❑	❑	❑
I have blurred or double vision	❑	❑	❑	❑	❑	❑
I have insomnia or other sleep problems	❑	❑	❑	❑	❑	❑
I have difficulty concentrating	❑	❑	❑	❑	❑	❑
My mood changes suddenly	❑	❑	❑	❑	❑	❑
I am anxious or nervous	❑	❑	❑	❑	❑	❑
I have outbursts of temper	❑	❑	❑	❑	❑	❑
I feel disoriented	❑	❑	❑	❑	❑	❑
I have trouble making decisions	❑	❑	❑	❑	❑	❑
I am forgetful	❑	❑	❑	❑	❑	❑
	Always	Often	Some-times	Never		
My symptoms disappear after I eat ...	❑	❑	❑	❑		

Hypoglycemia Workbook

Think about the changes you have seen in your health so far. You have filled in the Checklist, but what about other benefits?

As I worked through getting my own hypoglycemia under control, I noticed that my hypoglycemia symptoms were becoming less severe and less frequent, but there were also benefits I didn't expect. My weight started to drop steadily and my hormone related symptoms and my allergy symptoms were improving. I also noticed that I wasn't as moody and I was much easier to get along with, at least partly because my sleep was improving.

Are you starting to see benefits like these? Think about how you are feeling now. Check your first Food Journal and compare it to your most recent Food Journal. Is it noticeably different? Consider how you felt when you started this workbook. Are there things that you are able to do now that your symptoms wouldn't allow before? Write down any changes you have noticed in the space below.

_____

_____

_____

_____

_____

_____

You may want to wait a few weeks to let yourself settle into your new habits before making any more changes. When you are ready to continue your improvement, proceed to Step 7.

Step 7 — Find the hidden sugars

Many people with hypoglycemia cannot tolerate even low levels of sugar. If you are still experiencing symptoms, you will have to look for the hidden sugar in your diet.

For the next few weeks, read the labels of everything you buy and watch for the hidden sugars listed on page 143. I call these sugars "hidden" because they aren't always listed with names that make it obvious that they are nothing more than sugar.

Keep in mind that hidden sugars also include naturally occurring sugars like the fructose in all fruit and the lactose in milk and milk products. Sometimes food labels will show that the product contains 0 grams of sugar, but this just means added sugar. For example, canned fruit, even when it is packed in juice rather than sweetened syrup, still contains sugar. Even naturally occurring sugars can cause hypoglycemic symptoms.

Consider this excerpt from a recent article on the CBC Marketplace website:

> Our sweet tooth sure isn't lost on the makers of processed foods—every year they pour more sugars into more products. Statistics Canada has some numbers on how much we eat - about 23 teaspoons of added sugars everyday.
>
> But that only includes refined sugars and honey and maple syrup. Those 23 teaspoons don't include all the other added sugars we get from corn sweeteners—the main ingredient in pop. And, they don't include the sugars in fruit juices.

www.cbc.ca/consumers/market/files/food/sugar/

Hypoglycemia Workbook

Many "sugar-free" products that you will find on the shelves also contain hidden sugars. Instead of being sweetened with sugar, many "sugar-free" jams and jellies, for instance, are sweetened with fruit juice, often grape.

Whether you get your sugar from the sugar bowl or from grape juice, the effect on your body is the same and if you are hypoglycemic, you are likely to have unpleasant symptoms when you eat it.

Reading Labels

In addition to finding out what the ingredients are, we can also find out (approximately) how much of each ingredient there is in the package. The ingredients are listed in order by the amount in which they exist in the recipe (by weight). The food product contains more of the top ingredient than the second one, and more of the third ingredient than the one that appears fourth on the list. Review the label-reading section on page 116.

Reading labels is going to be your most important new skill and it is not difficult to do. Check every label for the following:

▌ What are the first 3 ingredients on the list? If any of these is sugar or a hidden sugar from the list on page 143, put the package back on the shelf and s-l-o-w-l-y back away!

▌ Consider what you would use if you were to make this food yourself. Look at the top 4 or 5 ingredients. Are these ingredients that you have in your kitchen?

▌ Read the names of the chemicals that have been added. If

you can't even pronounce many of the ingredients, don't buy the product.

Only the first point above is directly related to your hypoglycemia, but if you have food sensitivities, they will be easier to pinpoint if you have eliminated most chemicals.

Download the list of the names of the hidden sugars from www.theOtherSugarDisease.com and use it when you are shopping. Check the labels of everything you pick up in the grocery store for these ingredients. To really eliminate sugar from your diet, you need to eliminate these, too.

Practice reading labels and work on eliminating hidden sugars. Start by doing this for several weeks. This has four benefits.
1. You will learn to identify hidden sugars,
2. Reading labels will become a habit,
3. Your body will continue getting used to being sugar free, and
4. You will continue to learn what you can eat to feel better.

After a few weeks of reducing or eliminating hidden sugars, go to Step 8 to use the Symptom Checklist one more time.

Shop the perimeter of the store and stay away from the aisles that have the over-processed packaged foods.

Step 8 — One more check

You have worked hard over the last few weeks and you have learned how to eat well to feel your best. When you feel ready, take this symptom survey one more time. This should show just how far you have come.

If you are still experiencing severe or incapacitating symptoms, or if you haven't seen significant improvement, please visit your doctor. You may have underlying problems that need treatment other than a change in diet.

If, in doing this one last survey, you found that you are experiencing fewer symptoms and they are appearing less often, Congratulations! You are learning how to live well with hypoglycemia! Please write me at anita@theOther SugarDisease.com. I would love to hear your story.

Join your co-workers for lunch instead of eating at your desk. You'll enjoy your meal more and you'll get in the socializing you may miss when you start skipping cigarette breaks.

Symptom Checklist

	Frequency			Severity		
	Daily	Weekly	Monthly	Mild	Moderate	Severe
My heart races	❏	❏	❏	❏	❏	❏
I am irritable before eating (better after I eat)	❏	❏	❏	❏	❏	❏
I tremble or feel shaky	❏	❏	❏	❏	❏	❏
I suddenly start sweating	❏	❏	❏	❏	❏	❏
I feel clammy all over	❏	❏	❏	❏	❏	❏
I feel like I am trembling inside	❏	❏	❏	❏	❏	❏
I feel nauseous	❏	❏	❏	❏	❏	❏
My hands and feet are cold	❏	❏	❏	❏	❏	❏
I am constantly hungry	❏	❏	❏	❏	❏	❏
I feel mentally "cloudy"	❏	❏	❏	❏	❏	❏
My pupils are dilated	❏	❏	❏	❏	❏	❏
I feel faint	❏	❏	❏	❏	❏	❏
I feel apprehensive	❏	❏	❏	❏	❏	❏
I am tired	❏	❏	❏	❏	❏	❏
I have headaches or migraines	❏	❏	❏	❏	❏	❏
I feel dizzy	❏	❏	❏	❏	❏	❏
I have blurred or double vision	❏	❏	❏	❏	❏	❏
I have insomnia or other sleep problems	❏	❏	❏	❏	❏	❏
I have difficulty concentrating	❏	❏	❏	❏	❏	❏
My mood changes suddenly	❏	❏	❏	❏	❏	❏
I am anxious or nervous	❏	❏	❏	❏	❏	❏
I have outbursts of temper	❏	❏	❏	❏	❏	❏
I feel disoriented	❏	❏	❏	❏	❏	❏
I have trouble making decisions	❏	❏	❏	❏	❏	❏
I am forgetful	❏	❏	❏	❏	❏	❏
	Always	Often	Some-times	Never		
My symptoms disappear after I eat ...	❏	❏	❏	❏		

Sources

Adams, Junius. 2003. "Orthomolecular Psychiatry" [online]. [cited 13 July, 2003]. Available from: www.schizophrenia.org/ortho.html.

Agatston, Arthur. *The South Beach Diet*. New York: Rodale, 2003

Airola, Dr. Paavo. *Hypoglycemia: A Better Approach*. Phoenix: Health Plus, Publishers, 1984

Angell, Jenefer (Managing Editor). "Ménière's Disease" [online]. *HealthNotes*. [cited 13 July, 2003]. Available from: www.my custompak.com/healthNotes/Concern/Menieres_Disease.htm

Arrowsmith, Anne. "Hypoglycemia" [online]. [cited 12 July, 2003]. Available from: www.valiant50015.free serve.co.uk/Hypoglycemia3.html

Atkins, Robert. C., M.D. *Dr. Atkins New Diet Revolution*. New York: M. Evans and Company, 2002

Brand-Miller, Jennie Ph.D., Thomas M.S. Wolever, M.D., Ph.D., Stephen Colagiuri, M.D., Kaye Foster-Powell, M.Nutr. & Diet. *The Glucose Revolution*. New York: Marlowe & Company, 1999

Burkett, Glenn. "Chronic Fatigue / Energy" [online]. [cited 29 July, 2002]. Available from: www.glennburkett.com/chronic_fatigue.htm

Burkett, Glenn. "Fibromylagia" [online]. [cited 29 July, 2003]. Available from: www.glennburkett.com/fibromyalgia.htm

Cabot, Sandra, M.D. "Aspartame Makes You Fatter" [online]. [cited 13 July, 2003]. Available from: www.aspartamekills.com/aspartam.htm

Chapin, Barrett M.D. "Understanding Hypoglycemia" [online]. Compuserve Discussion. [cited 12 July, 2003]. Available from: www.fred.net/slowup/hcauses.txt

Chase, Dr. Jennifer. Northwest Nazarene University [online]. "Chapter 23: Gluconeogenesis and Glycogen Metabolism", [cited 11 July, 2003]. Available from: www.courses.nnu.edu/cm342jc/powerpoint/ch23a.ppt

Cleave, T.L. *The Saccharine Disease*. New Canaan, Connecticut: Keats, 1975

Cohen, Elizabeth. "Fat Chance." Cable News Network [aired July 6, 2002]

Constable, Debbie. "Fructose Intolerance, Hereditary" [online] The GAP Index. [cited 12 July, 2003]. Available from: www.icomm.ca/geneinfo/fructint.htm

Cosford, Robyn, MB, BS (Hons), FACNEM. "Insulin Resistance, Obesity and Diabetes: The Connection", *Journal of Australian College of Nutritional & Environmental Medicine* Vol 18 No 1, April 1999

Crook, William G., M.D. "Candida: The Hidden Disease", *Alive: Canadian Journal of Health and Nutrition* #225, July 2001

Debe, Dr. Joseph A. "A Natural Approach to Treating Depression" [online]. Available from: [cited 13 July, 2003]. www.drdebe.com/DEPRESS1.htm

Diabetes Dictionary [online]. [cited 12 July, 2003]. Available from: www.childrenwithdiabetes.com/dictionary/k.htm

Diabetic Guide. "High-Fiber Grains Protect Against Diabetes" [online]. [cited 12 July, 2003]. Available from: www.diabeticguide.com/diabetic guide/articles/artical_highfibergrains.htm

Ford-Martin, Paula. "Insulin Resistance on the Rise in Kids" [online]. [cited 10 July, 2002]. Available from: www.diabetes.about.com/library/blnews/blnHHSkidsobesity302.htm

Francis, Raymond. "Sugar is Killing Our Children" [online]. Beyond Health News. [cited 12 July, 2003]. Available from: www.beyond health.com/articles/Sugar_Killing_Our_Children.pdf

Giedt, Frances Towner and B. Polin, Ph.D. "Type II Diabetes and Syndrome X" [online]. [cited 10 July, 2002]. Available from: www.diabetic-lifestyle.com/articles/jun00_whats_1.htm

GNC Health Notes, "Insulin Resistance Syndrome", [online]. [cited 13 August, 2002]. Available from: www.gnc.com/health_notes/Concern/Insulin_Resistance_Syndrome.htm

GNC Health Notes. "Vitamin Guide" [online]. [cited 6 August, 2002]. Available from: www.gnc.com/health_notes/

Great Smokies Diagnostic Laboratories. "Depression and Glucose/Insulin" [online]. [cited 13 July, 2003]. Available from: www.gsdl.com/assessments/finddisease/depression/glucose_insulin.html

Hart, Cheryle, R. M.D., Mary Kay Grossman, R.D. *The Insulin Resistance Diet*. Chicago, Illinois: McGraw-Hill, 2001

HealthandAge.com. "Supplements" [online]. [cited 29 July, 2002]. Available from: www.healthandage.com/html/res/com/ConsLookups/Supplements.html

Heather, Cary, Simona Heather. "Korean Ginseng" [online]. [cited 28 July, 2003]. Available from: www.zooscape.com/cgi-bin/maitred/GreenCanyon?quest=r100045&proclivity=express&specie=US

Hill, Jim, Ph.D. University of Colorado, National Weight Control Registry [online]. [cited 12 July, 2003]. Available from: www.lifespan.org/services/bmed/wt_loss/nwcr/

Hill, John, M.D. "Nutritional Therapy for Thyroid Health and Hypothyroid Support" [online]. [cited 13 July, 2003]. Available from: www.advance-health.com/HypoThyroid.html

Hoffman, Dr. Ronald L. "Nicotine Dependency and Smoking Cessation" [online]. [cited 13 July, 2003]. Available from: www.drhoffman.com/jodinovember/

Holistic-online.com. "Herbs for Diabetes" [online]. [cited 30 July, 2002]. Available from: www.holistic-online.com/Remedies/Diabetes/diabetes_herbs.htm

Hypoglycemia and Supplement information [online]. [cited 6 August, 2002]. Available from: (http:// go-symmetry.com

Hypoglycemia Association Bulletin #44 [online]. [cited 13 July, 2003]. Available from: www.fred.net/slowup/ habul44.html)

Hurd, Karen. "Meniere's Syndrome" [online]. [cited 13 July, 2003]. Available from: www.nutrition-help.com/Health_ Concerns_Meniere's_Syndrome.htm

Insulin Resistance (Dysmetabolic) Syndrome Conference Statement of Purpose. 2002 [online]. [cited 10 August, 2002]. Available from: www.aace.com/pub/BMI/ purpose.php

Iridology Research "The Pancreas" [online]. [cited 12 July, 2003]. Available from: www.iridologyresearch.com/pages/Studies/study/Pancreas/page1.htm

Josephs, Allen S., M.D. "Vitacost Nutrient Guide Index" [online]. [cited 13 July, 2003]. Available from: www.vitacost.com/science/hn/hn70db/healthnotes/healthnote_2461007.html#C

Krimmel, Patricia, Edward Krimmel and Patricia T Krimmel. *The Low Blood Sugar Cookbook*. Bryn Mawr, PA: Franklin Publishers, 1986

Light, Marilyn. *Hypoglycemia: One of the most widespread and misdiagnosed diseases*. New Canaan, Connecticut: Keats Publishing Inc., 1983

Marks, Jennifer B. M.D. "The Insulin Resistance Syndrome" [online]. University of Miami School of Medicine. [cited 12 July, 2003]. Available from: (www.woundcare.org/newsvol1n3/ar1.htm

Mathews-Larson, Joan PhD, CCDP. "Hypoglycemia and Alcoholism" [online]. [cited 12 July, 2003]. Available from: www.healthrecovery.com/alcoholism_hypoglycemia.html

MayoClinic.com. "Ketotic Hypoglycemia" [online]. [cited 12 July, 2003]. Available from: www.ohiohealth.com/healthreference/reference/46CE30AC-C117-43EFA083821EFED99153.htm?category=questions

MayoClinic.com. "Hypoglycemia" [online]. [cited 12 July, 2003]. Available from: www.ohiohealth.com/healthreference/reference/ 69EA49D2-EA38-4A8A-95DB164A2555B514.htm? category=diseases

McArthur, John D. "Carbohydrates Fuel Your Brain" [online]. [cited 11 July, 2003]. Available from: www.fi.edu/brain/nutrition/ carbohydrates/index.html

Mead, Patricia. BA "Section 5—Glucose Tolerance" [online]. [cited 6 August, 2002]. Available from: www.askthehealthnuts.com/ answer5.htm

MedAngel.com. 2001. "Everything you always wanted to know about Sugar" [online]. [cited 11 July, 2003]. Available from: www.substance.altmedangel.com/sugar.htm

MedAngel.com. "The Truth About Diabetes" [online]. [cited 8 October, 2002]. Available from: www.illness.altmedangel.com/diabetes.htm

Medicinal Herbs Online. "Hypoglycemia" [online]. [cited 6 August, 2002]. Available from: www.egreg ore.com/diseases/hypogly cemia.html

Medline Plus, Medical Encyclopedia. "Infant of Diabetic Mother" [online]. [cited 12 July, 2003]. Available from: www. nlm.nih.gov/ medlineplus/ency/article/001597.htm

Mendosa, Rick. [online]. [cited October, 2002]. Available from: www.mendosa.com

Mendosa, Rick. "Revised International Table of Glycemic Index (GI) and Glycemic Load (GL) Values—2002" [online]. [cited 13 July, 2003]. Available from: www.members. lycos.co.uk/ramendosa/gilists.htm

Mennen, Barry, M.D. "Dietary Chromium: An Overview" [online]. [cited 24 July, 2002]. Available from: www.mineraltoddy.com/resinfo/ introchrom.htm

Mercola, Dr. Joseph. 2003. "Lower Your Grains & Lower Your Insulin Levels! A Novel Way To Treat Hypoglycemia" [online]. [cited 11 July, 2003]. Available from: www.mercola.com/article/Diet/ carbohydrates/lower_your_grains.htm

Merriam Webster Medical Dictionary [online]. [cited 11 July, 2003]. Available from: www.Inteli Health.com

MotherNature.com. "Hypoglycemia" [online]. [cited 13 July, 2003]. Available from: www.mothernature.com/Library/ Ency/index.cfm ?id=1034003

National Headache Foundation "Hypoglycemia" [online]. [cited 13 July, 2003]. Available from: www.headaches.org/consumer/ topicsheets/ hypoglycemia.html

National Institutes of Health [online]. "Selenium." [cited 7 August, 2002]. Available from: www.health link.mcw.edu/article/964647329.html

Network for Optimal Aging and Wellness News [online]. "Insulin Resistance." [cited 11 July, 2003]. Available from: www.noaw.com /Insulin%20Resistance/insulin.htm

Newman, Freda, RNC [online]. [cited 8 August, 2002]. Available from: www.fredacare.com

Nieves, Myrna R. M.D. FAAP. "Hypoglycemia in the Infant and Child" [online]. [cited 12 July, 2003]. Available from: www.home.coqui.net/ myrna/hypog.htm

Paada, Sukhdeep, M.D. "Dumping Syndrome" [online]. eMedicine. [cited 12 July, 2003]. Available from: www.emedicine.com/ med/topic589.htm

Page, Linda, N.D. Ph.D. "World of Healthy Healing: Ginseng" [online]. [cited 8 August, 2002]. Available from: www.healthyhealing.com/ GNS-KindsOfGinseng.html

Plesman, Jurriaan, BA (Psych). "The Forgotten Factor In The Crime Debate" [online]. Post Graduate Diploma Clinical Nutrition. [cited 12 July, 2003]. Available from: www.hypoglycemia.asn.au/ articles/forgotten_factor_crimedebate.html

Prevention.com [online]. "Insulin Resistance Syndrome: The New Silent Killer." [cited 12 July, 2003]. Available from: www. prevention.com/ cda/feature2002/0,4780,4085,00.html

Punjab Agricultural University. [online]. "The Art of Health: Enzymes – The Body's Structural Levels." [cited 6 August, 2002]. Available from: www. pua.edu/peter1/chapter_16c.htm

Rall, Judie C. "Biotin: For Great Hair and Nails" [online]. [cited 14 August, 2002]. Available from: www.unhinderedliving.com/ biotin.html

Raloff, Janet. "The New GI Tracks" [online]. Science News (internet edition), April 8th, 2000. [cited 12 July, 2003]. Available from: www.findarticles.com/cf_dls/m1200/15_157/62052385/p1 /article.jhtml

Reaven, Gerald, M.D., Terry Kristen Strom, M.B.A. and Barry Fox, Ph.D. *Syndrome X: Overcoming the Silent Killer That Can Give You a Heart Attack.* New York: Simon and Schuster, 2000.

Sources

Rosalyn's Healthy Lifestyles. "Hypoglycemia." Rosalyn's Healthy Lifestyles [online]. [cited 29 July, 2002]. Available from: www.rosalynshealthylifestyles.com/HealthBaskets/hypoglycemia.htm

Rosedale, Ron, M.D. "Insulin and its Metabolic Effects". Designs for Health Institute 1999 [online]. [cited 12 July, 2003]. Available from: www.dfhi.com/interviews/rosedale.html

Rosedale, Ron, M.D. "Nutrition for Health: An Introduction to the Proper Diet." International Center for Metabolic and Longevity Medicine, 2003

Rosedale, Ron and Carol Coleman. *The Rosedale Diet*. New York: HarperCollins Publishers, Inc., 2004

Rosenthal, Norman, M.D. (Reviewer). "Seasonal Affective Disorder." National Institute of Mental Health, May 1998 [online]. [cited 13 July, 2003]. Available from: www.ocd.nami.org/helpline/sad.htm

Rogers, Lois. "Low-fat diet may pile on weight". *Sunday Times/London* [online]. [cited 13 July, 2003]. Available from: www.universaltao.co.uk/lowfat.htm

Roth, Ronald. "MIGRAINE / HEADACHES: Nutritional Causes, Prevention and Therapies" [online]. [cited 13 July, 2003]. Available from: www.acu-cell.com/dis-hea.html

Saunders, Jeraldine and Harvey M., Ross M.D. *Hypoglycemia: The Disease Your Doctor Won't Treat*. New York: Kensington Publishing Corp, 1980

Salisbury University."Ginseng". A Nurses Guide to Herbal Remedies [online]. [cited 7 August, 2002]. Available from: www.salisbury.edu/Schools/Henson/NursingDept/Herbalremedies/ginseng.htm

Sangsters Vitamin and Mineral Reference Chart [online]. [cited 14 August, 2002]. Available from: www.sangsters.com/charts.shtml

Schmidt, Darren, D.C., N.D. "Modern Food Trends". Wholistic Doctor [online]. [cited 12 July, 2003]. Available from: www.wholisticdoc.com/index/19

Schorr, Melissa. "Many diabetics unaware of their heart disease risk" [online], Reuters Health 2002-06-18 [cited 12 July, 2003]. Available from: www.12.42.224.156/health news/reuters/NewsStory 0618200224.htm

Schwarzbein, Diana, M.D. *The Schwarzbein Principle II*. Deerfield Beach, Florida: Health Communications Inc., 2002

Sears, Barry, Ph. D. *The Zone*. New York: Harper Collins Regan Books, 2000

Shiel, Dr. William, M.D., Chief Medical Editor. "Hypoglycemia" [online]. [cited 12 July, 2003]. Available from: www.medicinenet.com/ Hypoglycemia/page3.htm

Shomon, Mary. "How to Tell If You Are Hypothyroid" [online]. [cited 13 July, 2003]. Available from: www.thyroid.about.com/ library/howto/hthypothyroidism.htm

Smith Waddel, Rebecca. "PCOS Frequently Asked Questions" [online]. [cited 13 July, 2003]. Available from: www.inciid.org/faq/ pcos.html

Starlanyl, Devin M.D. "Reactive Hypoglycemia (RHG): FM/MPS Perpetuating Factor" [online]. [cited 12 July, 2003]. Available from: www.tidalweb.com/ fms/rhg.shtml

Tenney, Louise, M.H. *Hypoglycemia: A Nutritional Approach.* Pleasant Grove, UT: Woodland Publishing, Inc., 1996

The American Holistic Medical Association [online]. [cited 13 July, 2003]. Available from: www.holisticmedicine.org

The Merck Manual of Diagnosis and Therapy. "Gastrointestinal Disorders" [online]. [cited 12 July, 2003]. Available from: www.merck.com/pubs/mmanual/section3/chapter34/ 34e.htm

The Way Up Newsletter. "Benefits of Amino Acid, L-Glutamine" [online]. [cited 7 August, 2002]. Available from: www.thewayup.com/ newsletters/041501.htm

The Way Up Newsletter. "Pancreatin" [online]. [cited 6 August, 2002]. Available from: www.thewayup.com/ newsletters/041501.htm

The Way Up Newsletter. Vol 15 12/15/99 [online]. [cited 13 August, 2002]. Available from: (www.thewayup.com/ newsletters/121599.htm

Tinnerello, Donna, MS, RD, CD/N. "Hypoglycemia" [online]. [cited 12 July, 2003]. Available from: www.alwaysyourchoice.com/ayc/ nutrition/diet_disease/hypoglycemia.php

Tinnerello, Donna, MS, RD, CD/N. "Irritable Bowel Syndrome" [online]. June 2000. [cited 13 July, 2003]. Available from: www.always yourchoice.com/ayc/nutrition/diet_disease/ibs_nutri.php

Tourette Syndrome Foundation of Canada. *Understanding Tourette Syndrome: A Handbook for Educators.* Toronto: Tourette Syndrome Foundation of Canada, 2001

Wart, Paula J. "Glycemic Load Explained" [online]. [cited 13 July, 2003]. Available from: www.vanderbiltowc.wellsource.com/dh/con tent.asp?ID=655

Weller, Charles, M.D. and Brian Richard Boylan. *How to Live with Hypoglycemia*. New York: Doubleday & Company, 1984

Whitworth, Claudia. "What is PCOS" [online]. [cited 13 July, 2003]. Available from: www.pcos.net/ whatis.html

Wilson, Dr. "New Information about Yeast Infections" [online]. [cited 29 July, 2002]. Available from: www.drwilson.com.articles/ candidafungus.htm

Wolfe, Lynne A., MS, PNP, BC. "Carbohydrate Metabolism and Blood Sugar Monitoring" [online]. [cited 11 July, 2003]. Available from: www.fodsupport.org/ blood_sugar_monitoring.htm

Wurges, Jennifer. "Brewer's Yeast" [online]. *Gale Encyclopedia of Alternative Medicine*. [cited 27 July, 2002]. Available from: www.findarticles.com

Young, David G., N.D. "Minerals" [online]. [cited 27 July, 2002]. Available from: www.angelfire.com/ nd/drdavid/minerals.html)

Zeischegg, Dr. Peter M. "Hypoglycemia" [online]. [cited 13 July, 2003]. Available from: www.drz.org/asp/conditions/hypogly cemia2.asp)

Some Resources for You

Hypoglycemia organizations

Here are some helpful hypoglycemia organizations that are accessible on the Internet. Each of these sites include lots of useful information, but none have been updated recently.

The Hypoglycemia Health Organization of Australia

www.hypoglycemia.asn.au—This website has information about symptoms, diagnosis and even includes a letter you can take to your doctor to help explain hypoglycemia and how to order and interpret glucose tolerance testing.

The Hypoglycemia Support Foundation, Inc.

www.hypoglycemia.org—Founded and run by Roberta Ruggiero, this website sells a Hypoglycemia Survival Kit which includes:

The Do's and Don'ts of Low Blood Sugar: An Everyday Guide to Hypoglycemia by Roberta Ruggiero

The Blood Sugar Hotline—a 45-minute audiotape about a journey with hypoglycemia

HSF Today—a one-year subscription to their quarterly newsletter

The Health Emergency Card—a wallet card to identify you as a hypoglycemic for use in emergency treatment situations

Hypoglycemia Homepage Holland

www.lightning.prohosting.com/~hypoglyc/—This site includes a great deal of useful information about hypoglycemia symptoms, although the constant advertising by the website host gets annoying after a while.

Web sites

There is an abundance of information about hypoglycemia on the internet. Many sites concentrate on hypoglycemia in diabetics but there is also quite a lot of information about reactive hypoglycemia and insulin resistance. Some useful sites include:

www.mercola.com—Dr. Mercola is one of the most quoted of the doctors treating hypoglycemia.

www.mendosa.com—This one includes comprehensive Glycemic Index lists.

www.fred.net/slowup/habul44.html—This site has lots of information about hypoglycemia symptoms.

www.everythingatkins.net—This is the official Atkins web site. Lots of information about low carbohydrate eating here.

www.radiantrecovery.com—This site is particularly useful for people just getting started with hypoglycemia, and this is where I got the idea for a step-by-step approach for dietary change.

www.sugarshock.com—This is a fun and informative site for helping people "kick sugar". Connie Benesch, Managing Editor of the site, is also the founder and moderator of the Yahoo KickSugar on-line group.

Internet hypoglycemia groups

There are also some good hypoglycemia groups on the web. You can get a lot of helpful information and advice from other hypoglycemics. Two good examples I know of are Yahoo groups called *hypo* and *kicksugar* respectively. There is also a *lowcarbmealplanning* group on msn.com

What readers are saying about *Hypoglycemia: The Other Sugar Disease.*

Just wanted to say thanks for the email....it helps to be reminded that there are others out there with hypoglycemia too. I just start to get going with the diet and I end up cheating!! But I keep going back and trying some more. So, I hope that soon I will be following the diet perfectly. Your book and information helped me immensely. I, like many of us was unwell for a VERY long time before figuring out what was wrong. So just wanted to say thanks for the email and for getting a book out there that can help so many people.

Sincerely, Heather

I just wanted to let you know that I am so blessed to have found you; you have been such a help and inspiration to me. Your book has been very helpful on leading me back into good health. I started eating the way I should be around 3 weeks ago. I'm no longer craving big servings of food on my breaks and lunch at work like I was. I am now eating just a bit of fruit and a handful of all natural almonds or sunflower kernels on my breaks and a salad with either egg or deli meats or with just nuts sprinkled in. I vary that some; I even like a little cottage cheese mixed in. And for dinner, I eat fresh or frozen vegetables, with chicken or fish. Salmon is my favorite. I'm quickly discovering that by cutting way back portion-wise and eating frequently, I'm getting less headaches and less feeling miserably starving. It's a great feeling.

Thanks, Susan S.

I sent off for your book and it has become my bible. It is written in layman's language and I re-read it every few weeks. As I go along I am picking up new tips all the time. I have more good days than bad days now and when I have a bad day I am able to work out why. Along the way I have found out that caffeine has caused the 30 years of bad headaches (I haven't had any since I went caffeine free in May, apart from one cup of tea a week after I stopped and I ended up with a 24 hour migraine!), and potatoes leave me comatose about one half hour after a meal. I haven't lost any weight yet but I am trying to concentrate on health not weight but in the last week have realised that if I cut rice and pasta from my evening meal and stick to proteins before bed my weight has stabilised instead of going up so I am hopeful of a possible weight loss soon.

Many thanks for your book—it so helps to know that there is a solution and I can do something about it myself. I have become very disillusioned with doctors over recent years—hitting 40 does not automatically turn a woman neurotic or panic-stricken, she may actually have something wrong with her!

Linda M.

Feedback about the website — www.anitaflegg.com — and Anita's Weekly Hypoglycemia Survival Tips.

I came across your website which I found to be not only interesting but very educational. I only wish my doctor would have described hypoglycemia the way you did and I would have understood what was wrong with me all along. Your website made a lot of sense!! That's exactly how I felt for the past 2 years and it wasn't until I drastically changed my diet and totally cut down on my high carbs and sugar intake that I started feeling a whole lot better!! I want to thank you for your informative website. It made me realize that I was not alone and that I wasn't losing it mentally either.

Sincerely, Lis R.

I got more out of your webpage than I did out of all my doctor visits.

Tracey M.

Your emails and information are very beneficial. A lot of people, including medical professionals and even loved ones, are unfamiliar with our condition and don't always understand what we are going through: physically, physiologically, mentally, and emotionally. Your information has been a "blessing" to me.

Again, thanks. Larry J.

I've just read the last article on your Hypoglycemia website and wanted to send you a well deserved pat on the back. I've read many websites, books and publications on the subject. In my opinion, yours has the most accurate information and is superbly articulated.

The quote in your material that helped me the most was the one referring to a Ferrari and premium fuel. I've always thought there was something wrong with me because I could not eat dessert (like my peers) without suffering fatigue. Your quality information has helped me form a better perspective on diet, and for that I thank you sincerely.

Michael

You have written information on hypoglycemia on your web site that has helped clarify some issues for me on this. You write well, clearly, and your perspective is my perspective: what is going on with my body and why??!! So you answer questions without my even having to ask them. Thank you for your generosity in writing down what you know logically and clearly. It is of inestimable value to someone such as me who's searching for answers to why I have hypoglycemia. And since the hypoglycemia adds to the feeling of panic, your web site is a very welcome and calming.

Thank you again. Roxanne